The Aging Population in the Twenty-First Century

Statistics for Health Policy

Dorothy M. Gilford, Editor

Panel on Statistics for an Aging Population
Sam Shapiro, Chair

Committee on National Statistics
Commission on Behavioral and Social Sciences and Education
National Research Council

NATIONAL ACADEMY PRESS
Washington, D.C. 1988

National Academy Press • 2101 Constitution Avenue, N.W. • Washington, D. C. 20418

NOTICE: The project that is the subject of this report was approved by the Governing Board of the National Research Council, whose members are drawn from the councils of the National Academy of Sciences, the National Academy of Engineering, and the Institute of Medicine. The members of the committee responsible for the report were chosen for their special competences and with regard for appropriate balance.

This report has been reviewed by a group other than the authors, according to procedures approved by a Report Review Committee consisting of members of the National Academy of Sciences, the National Academy of Engineering, and the Institute of Medicine.

The National Academy of Sciences is a private, nonprofit, self-perpetuating society of distinguished scholars engaged in scientific and engineering research, dedicated to the furtherance of science and technology and to their use for the general welfare. Upon the authority of the charter granted to it by the Congress in 1863, the Academy has a mandate that requires it to advise the federal government on scientific and technical matters. Dr. Frank Press is president of the National Academy of Sciences.

The National Academy of Engineering was established in 1964, under the charter of the National Academy of Sciences, as a parallel organization of outstanding engineers. It is autonomous in its administration and in the selection of its members, sharing with the National Academy of Sciences the responsibility for advising the federal government. The National Academy of Engineering also sponsors engineering programs aimed at meeting national needs, encourages education and research, and recognizes the superior achievements of engineers. Dr. Robert M. White is president of the National Academy of Engineering.

The Institute of Medicine was established in 1970 by the National Academy of Sciences to secure the services of eminent members of appropriate professions in the examination of policy matters pertaining to the health of the public. The Institute acts under the responsibility given to the National Academy of Sciences by its congressional charter to be an adviser to the federal government and, upon its own initiative, to identify issues of medical care, research, and education. Dr. Samuel O. Thier is president of the Institute of Medicine.

The National Research Council was organized by the National Academy of Sciences in 1916 to associate the broad community of science and technology with the Academy's purposes of furthering knowledge and advising the federal government. Functioning in accordance with general policies determined by the Academy, the Council has become the principal operating agency of both the National Academy of Sciences and the National Academy of Engineering in providing services to the government, the public, and the scientific and engineering communities. The Council is administered jointly by both Academies and the Institute of Medicine. Dr. Frank Press and Dr. Robert M. White are chairman and vice chairman, respectively, of the National Research Council.

This project was supported with funds from the Veterans Administration and six agencies of the U.S. Department of Health and Human Services: the Health Care Financing Administration, the National Center for Health Statistics, the National Institute of Mental Health, the National Institute on Aging, the Office of the Assistant Secretary for Planning and Evaluation, and the Social Security Administration.

Library of Congress Cataloging-in-Publication Data

National Research Council (U.S.). Panel on Statistics
    for an Aging Population.
    The aging population in the twenty-first century.

    Bibliography: p.
    1. Aged—Diseases—United States—Statistics.
2. Aged—Medical care—United States—Statistics.
3. Aged—Diseases—United States—Forecasting.
4. Health planning—United States. I. Gilford,
Dorothy M. II. Title. [DNLM: 1. Aged—United States—
Statistics. 2. Health Policy—United States.
3. Health services for the aged—United States.
WT 100 N2775a]
RA408.A3N37   362.1'9897'00973021   88-15151
ISBN 0-309-03881-2

Printed in the United States of America

First Printing, May 1988
Second Printing, November 1988

PANEL ON STATISTICS FOR AN AGING POPULATION

SAM SHAPIRO (*Chair*), Health Services Research and Development Center, Johns Hopkins University

DAN GERMAN BLAZER II, Department of Psychiatry, Duke University Medical Center

LAURENCE G. BRANCH, School of Public Health, Boston University

NEAL E. CUTLER, Department of Political Science, University of Southern California

JEANNE E. GRIFFITH, Congressional Research Service, Library of Congress

ROBERT LOUIS KAHN, Institute for Social Research, University of Michigan

GARY G. KOCH, Department of Biostatistics, University of North Carolina

JUDITH RICE LAVE, Graduate School of Public Health, University of Pittsburgh

KENNETH G. MANTON, Center for Demographic Studies, Duke University

DOROTHY P. RICE, Aging Health Policy Center, University of California, San Francisco

JOHN W. ROWE, Department of Gerontology, Harvard University

ETHEL SHANAS, Department of Sociology (emeritus), University of Illinois, Chicago

JAMES H. WARE, Department of Biostatistics, Harvard School of Public Health

DOROTHY M. GILFORD, *Study Director*
CAROLYN ROGERS, *Research Associate*
ANNE M. SPRAGUE, *Research Assistant*
LILLIAN GURALNICK, *Consultant*
THOMAS JABINE, *Consultant*
JANE TAKEUCHI, *Consultant*
CARLOTTA MOLITOR, *Administrative Secretary*

COMMITTEE ON NATIONAL STATISTICS

Contents

Preface

Concern about the aged has surfaced in recent years with such dramatic force and recognition by so many that the national response will have consequences far into the future, as has been true in past years. During the Great Depression, Old Age and Survivors Insurance (Social Security) was legislated to create a partnership of workers, employers, and government to make certain that income would not end for workers and their dependents simply because of advanced age. In 1965, after debates about national health insurance, Medicare was legislated to increase the access of the aged to health services by reducing economic barriers to care. While not as dramatic or comprehensive as these economic and health care measures, the Older Americans Act in 1965 and subsequent amendments opened the door to social and health-related programs that reach the elderly at the grass roots.

Today, the aged hold a central position in the preoccupation of policy makers in the legislative and executive branches of government about costs, organization, and quality of health services. This results from a conjunction of circumstances representing a mix of knowns and unknowns about the aged. We can describe with considerable certainty the growth of the elderly population that will follow from the present age composition of the population and the increases in life expectancy being experienced at every age, including the elderly. We also know that the need for institutional and noninstitutional health care and the related costs are high among the aged, generally, and that these increase substantially with advancing age.

But we are far from certain about the nature of the changes in health and functional status that may be under way among the aged, i.e., whether increases in longevity are associated mainly with longer periods of chronic illness and prolongation of dependency or with additional years of well-being and independent functioning. Furthermore, it is not certain how current and future policies designed to change the structure of the health care system and the costs and financing of health services affect access to care, the quality of care, and the quality of life for the elderly.

The issues involved are complex, but we are fortunate to have strong data systems that can be directed to meet the needs for information. This report is the product of a study that takes stock of specific questions faced in developing health policy for the elderly and charts a course for producing information from the existing national data systems to arrive at answers. The conclusions and recommendations represent the end point of a long process.

ORIGIN OF THE STUDY

The Panel on Statistics for an Aging Population was established in September 1984 under the aegis of the Committee on National Statistics and within the National Research Council to study the adequacy of current statistical information and methodology, particularly in the area of health and medical care, for an aging population. The panel's study is an outgrowth of an initiative throughout the National Academy of Sciences in aging begun in 1982 and coordinated by the Institute of Medicine. A standing committee, the Committee on an Aging Society, was established to develop a program of studies to address the major societal issues resulting from the changing demographics of the U.S. population.

In April 1983 the Academy complex sponsored a conference to determine whether the available statistics are adequate for policy analysis for the aging society or whether a study on this topic was warranted. The conference participants included representatives of several federal agencies and of organizations concerned with aging, congressional staff, and researchers on aging. The conferees identified a substantial number of problems with data on aging and strongly endorsed the need for a thorough study of the problems and the changes, large and small, that would increase the utility of national data systems. The task was seen as being of major proportions, and funding for a panel to study the issues was obtained from the Veterans Administration and six agencies of the Department of Health and Human Services: the Office of the Assistant Secretary for Planning and Evaluation, the National Center for Health Statistics, the National Institute on Aging, the National Institute of Mental Health, the Health Care Financing Administration, and the Social Security Administration. Panel members included individuals long experienced in health matters and drawn from many disciplines including statistics, health sciences, social sciences, and medicine (see Appendix F for biographical sketches).

EARLY PANEL ACTIVITIES

Panel members initially identified 12 issue areas relevant to the charge and commissioned experts in these areas to prepare background papers (Appendix A). These became working documents throughout our deliberations and were drawn on extensively in the preparation of this report. They represent significant contributions in themselves and will be published in a separate volume by the National Center for Health Statistics.

To identify data gaps, detailed knowledge of existing data sets was needed. The panel therefore developed a compilation of descriptions of available data sets relative to the health of the elderly, since existing inventories were out of date. The resulting volume, *Inventory of Data Sets Related to the Health of the Elderly*, describes 117 data sets and was published by the U.S. Senate Subcommittee on Aging in connection with the June 1986 Hearings on Statistical Policy for an Aging America.

To obtain advice from a wide range of experts and interested persons and organizations, the panel sponsored a one-day symposium in September 1985. The purpose of the symposium was to stimulate discussion about statistical problems encountered by policy makers and members of the research community in addressing issues concerned with an aging population. The panel's commissioned papers served as the focus of the symposium. More than 100 persons participated, including congressional staff, researchers on aging, and representatives from federal agencies, professional societies, and public interest groups.

CONCURRENT ACTIVITIES

During the course of the study, several major events related to the panel's charge took place. One was the Summit on Aging-Related Statistics, cosponsored by the National Institute on Aging and the Bureau of the Census, on May 2, 1986. The purpose of the summit was to determine how the federal statistical system can provide the data needed to answer policy questions for an aging society in a cost-efficient manner. To this end, participating agency directors prepared statements of their views of the vital issues regarding the elderly and agreed to establish an Interagency Forum on Aging-Related Statistics to encourage cooperation among the federal agencies in the development and coordination of data on the older population. Special attention was given to the areas of demography, epidemiology, health service utilization and costs, and socioeconomic characteristics of the elderly. The forum, now with multiagency participation, provides an important, ongoing mechanism for assessment by those targeted by the specific recommendations in this report and the measures needed to effect changes in data systems and in the production and analysis of information.

The other major event was a joint hearing on Statistical Policy for an Aging America held on June 3, 1986, by the Subcommittee on Aging of the U.S. Senate Committee on Labor and Human Resources and the Subcommittee on Energy, Nuclear Proliferation, and Government Processes of the U.S. Senate Committee on Governmental Affairs. The hearing examined the need to link data collection and research to planning and policy development, promote research coordination among the federal data collection agencies, and improve data accessibility, data quality, policy relevance, and the dissemination of aging-related statistics. The panel chair gave testimony on the concerns and preliminary conclusions of the panel.

A third related development is that a number of federal agencies have already taken steps to implement some of the panel's ideas—a fact that is not surprising, since in the course of the study some agency heads shared with the panel their long-range plans in a most beneficial interactive process. Staff members from the seven sponsoring agencies not only provided current information on agency activities, but also heard the panel discussions that led to the recommendations. In addition, staff from several agencies briefed us on plans for specific surveys; some of our recommendations are in fact our endorsement of aspects of these plans. Most of our recommendations regarding surveys are for continuing surveys; continuity remains an important aspect of the recommendations, even though we have evidence that the first implementation steps have been taken.

ACKNOWLEDGMENTS

The report as a whole represents contributions from every member of the panel. Many of the chapters were drafted and redrafted by panel members, and all chapters were subjected to detailed review at numerous sessions. The panel divided itself into working groups, which determined the structure and most of the substance of the report; the panel is particularly indebted to the chairs of the three working groups for their efforts. The Working Group on Health and Related Issues and Data Requirements, chaired by Daniel Blazer II, identified topics the panel should consider. The Working Group on Improvement of Data Resources for Policy Analysis of Aging, chaired by Dorothy Rice, developed the recommendations to fill the data gaps. The Working Group on Statistical Methodology for Health Policy Analysis, chaired by Gary Koch, took responsibility not only for the chapter on statistical methodology, but also for much of the material on health transitions and longitudinal studies found in other chapters.

The panel profited greatly from the perspectives provided by the liaison representatives of the seven federal agencies who sponsored the study; they were always ready to respond to questions raised by the panel. The liaison representatives, and in addition Jacob Feldman of the National Center for Health Statistics and Richard Suzman of the National Institute for Aging, deserve special thanks for their willingness to share with the panel their in-depth knowledge of health data and research related to the elderly. Early in the study, Leo Selker, who as a National Research Council fellow in residence at the Institute of Medicine, participated in the panel activities, contributed material for the demography chapter, and provided effective coordination with the Institute's activities related to the elderly. Joan Van Nostrand of the National Center for Health Statistics deserves our special appreciation not only for her management skill as monitor of a project complicated by multiple agency funding, but also, and more important, for her many contributions to the panel's activities and deliberations. Her advice and suggestions contributed significantly to the panel's report.

Our report also benefited from frequent dialogues with the Committee on National Statistics, which was chaired by Steven Fienberg during our study, and thoughtful comments from the reviewers for the committee as well as reviewers for the Commission on Behavioral and Social Sciences and Education. Burton Singer, the current chair of the committee, was particularly helpful in drafting material for the sections on designs and strategies for longitudinal data analysis for the chapter on statistical methodology. The panel appreciates the encouragement and administrative assistance received from Edwin D. Goldfield, director of the Committee on National Statistics while the study was under way, and from Miron Straf, the committee's director while the report was being prepared for publication. The report was markedly improved by the helpful suggestions made by Christine McShane, editor, and by the skillful reorganization of one chapter by Eugenia Grohman, associate director for reports, of the Commission on Behavioral and Social Sciences and Education.

The panel's support staff at the National Research Council was dedicated and effective. Thanks are due to Carolyn Rogers, who was on detail to the project staff from the Census Bureau for the first year of the study, during which she drafted material for the demography chapter; to Carlotta Molitor who, in addition to satisfying all the secretarial demands for a large study, handled the logistics for the symposium and the numerous meetings of the panel and its working groups; and to Anne Sprague, who managed the final stages of preparing the report for publication. Three consultants made special contributions to the report: Lillian Guralnick had primary responsibility for compiling the *Inventory of Data Sets Related to the Health of the Elderly* and also assisted in collecting information and redrafting parts of the report; Thomas Jabine prepared the section on record linkage; and Jane Takeuchi drafted much of the material on health promotion and disease prevention in addition to the material on health care expenditures.

The individual most responsible for originating the study and bringing it to a successful conclusion is Dorothy Gilford, the study director. Only an experienced hand could have overcome the difficulties a complex project of this type involves, and she had the wisdom, patience, and, in the end, the energy to bring the report to completion. Personally, and as chair of the panel, I am indebted to her.

Finally, I feel privileged to have had the opportunity to chair a panel that worked so well together and gave so much more time than could have been anticipated. I am confident that their efforts will have a lasting influence on the availability of information required to develop health policy and to evaluate the effect of the measures adopted.

Sam Shapiro, Chair
Panel on Statistics for
an Aging Population

1

Introduction and Summary of Recommendations

In the coming decade, the nation's decision makers will continue to be challenged by changing demands for social and health services due to the anticipated rapid rate of growth of the elderly (65 years or older) and especially the oldest-old (85 years or older) populations. In the 12 years until the year 2000, it is anticipated that the very old (80 years or older) U.S. population will be the largest single federal entitlement group, consuming $82.8 billion (1984 dollars) in benefits (Torrey, 1985). The growth of these populations will be even more rapid soon after the turn of the century, as the post World War II baby-boom cohorts become elderly.

To respond wisely to the multifaceted demands of an aging U.S. society, it is crucial to have the data and information necessary to make difficult choices about resource allocation and program structure. To produce this information: (1) appropriate data must be collected and (2) appropriate models and statistical methods must be applied to the analysis of those data. Although there is currently a sizable expenditure on data collection activities, the investment is minuscule compared with the size of the federal and state programs that this information is used to manage and direct. Furthermore, recent scientific evidence on the modifiable nature of health and functional transitions among the old and oldest-old populations suggests that many aspects of current data collection are inadequate to support policy analysis. Efforts dedicated to methodological development of improved analytic and forecasting tools are even more deficient. Data production and analysis, as well as methodological research, will need careful and thorough review, and modification in the light of that review, to maximize the utility of the data collected.

BACKGROUND

Concern about the inadequacies of statistical information and methodology available for policy decisions for the elderly is widespread. Seven federal agencies that shared this concern—the Veterans Administration and six agencies of the U.S. Department of Health and Human Services: the Health Care Financing Administration, the National Center for Health Statistics, the National Institute of Mental Health, the National Institute on Aging, the Office of the Assistant Secretary for Planning and Evaluation, and the Social Security Administration—joined forces and sponsored a study by the National Research Council to address these problems. The panel was charged with the following major activities:

1. To determine the data requirements for policy development for health care of the elderly during the next decade; to assess the statistical adequacy of current data sources pertaining to the health care of the elderly; and to identify major shortcomings and recommend appropriate remedies and actions;

2. To identify the essential components of a comprehensive program of statistics on the elderly that can be implemented within a decentralized statistical system (assuming continuation of the current decentralized system) and that would provide adequate data on aging for all functional areas and to recommend changes and procedures that would facilitate integrating data from the various components; and

3. To determine whether changes or refinements are needed in the statistical methodology used in health policy analysis or in the planning and administration of programs for the elderly and to recommend actions or further research.

The panel approached these charges in a period when budgetary constraints assumed special significance because of their implications for statistical activities of federal agencies. The panel therefore placed emphasis on modifications to existing national statistical programs and surveys and those that are getting under way—an approach that led to numerous recommendations but was designed to recognize current budget stringencies. Accordingly, the panel's recommendations, whenever possible, are formulated to capitalize on and enhance available data resources, surveys, and administrative records. Nevertheless, meeting the needs for data is not cost-free, and new budgetary support for existing agencies will be essential.

In making its recommendations, the panel has dealt with data requirements for the immediate future and has also provided a long-range planning guide for the collection and analysis of statistical data for policy analysis for the elderly population over the next decade. We recognize that many of the surveys and administrative record systems that are the subject of our recommendations are not limited to the elderly and that their implementation will have to fit into the agencies' comprehensive plans for improving their statistical systems. With careful planning, and some additional resources, it should be possible to implement all the recommendations before the twenty-first century. Several recommendations specify the frequency with which surveys should be conducted. The recommended cycles represent the best judgment of panel members, but we recognize that agencies will have to examine the proposed cycles more intensively, drawing on input from nongovernmental sources.

In the course of its work, the panel paid particular attention to overlap and duplication between the major data systems and concluded that data gaps are much more serious than overlap. There are surveys that appear to cover many of the same areas, but they differ substantially on specific components of concern to policy makers, particularly in content and the populations covered. Many of the data gaps are the result of program adjustments made by federal statistical agencies in response to the changing fiscal environment of the last decade and the accompanying reductions in budgetary support. In many cases, these changes were made hastily, without adequate consideration of their short-term and long-term consequences, and thus have not supported the development of information for well-informed public policy debate.

Because of budget reductions, the statistical agencies have been forced to make changes in programs and policies in recent years—changes that affect the availability of statistics on the elderly. These changes involve one or more of the following: (1) changing the focus from policy-oriented statistical programs to those that support the administrative aspects of government; (2) reducing the periodicity (or frequency of data collection) of major surveys; (3) reducing the coverage of surveys, through deletion of specific subpopulations from the universes of interest or through reduction of sample size;

(4) reducing efforts in the areas of data collection operations, data processing, and data dissemination; (5) reducing the timeliness of data dissemination, of both hard-copy reports and public-use data files; and (6) postponing or eliminating the regular review of data needs in developing areas, usually in the interest of protecting core programs within agencies. Specific examples of the types of adjustments cited above are considered in Appendix B, which examines the programs of those agencies responsible for the information bases used for supporting policy development in aging.

In short, the panel faced a complex task. Our deliberations took place during a cost-conscious era, there are serious gaps in the data needed for policy analysis, and we recognized the need to strike a balance between short- and long-term concerns in formulating our recommendations.

As a basis for its work the panel compiled an inventory (National Research Council, 1986) of 117 data sets related directly or indirectly to health of the elderly—data sets that remained following a decade of changes the agencies have been forced to make in response to budget stringency. Simply put, a systematic review of these data sets led the panel to the conclusion that the available information is inadequate for policy analysis. A major concern of the panel relates to remedying this situation and ensuring availability of information adequate in scope and timeliness for policy purposes. Careful attention has been paid to the most urgent improvements needed in the existing surveys and in the use that can be made of systems of administrative records. No new large information system is recommended: the panel considered it more cost-effective and more acceptable politically to obtain the new data required for policy use by adding to existing surveys. Recommendations in the report address data requirements that can be met by federal information systems that are national in coverage. The panel notes that data sets generated in epidemiological studies, longitudinal community surveys, and evaluation studies may be equally important for policy purposes, but they fall outside the scope of the charge of the panel.

HEALTH POLICY ISSUES

The Changing Policy Agenda

Changes in socioeconomic, demographic, and health care trends frequently raise new health policy issues. Other issues come to the attention of policy makers because of the efforts of interest groups and public officials or as a result of particular dramatic events. For example, the release of Medicare patients from hospitals who still require skilled nursing care with no provision for such care gave focus to concerns of the Senate Special Committee on Aging early in 1985 about the prospective payment system currently in use by the Medicare program. Such broad issues as the cost, the quality, or the availability of health care are continuously part of the general or systemic policy agenda of the country. When a particular issue becomes defined as a crisis, however, sufficient political interest may be generated to move alternative solutions to the more active policy agenda, where solutions are debated in the form of new legislation, appropriations, or regulations (Elder and Coble, 1984). Otherwise the issue will disappear from the policy agenda, although it may well reemerge on the active agenda with changes in the economic or political climate.

For example, in the 1970s the level and trend of national expenditures for health care moved cost containment and payment for health care to the top of the active policy agenda. In fact, in the late 1970s, the two major policy initiatives of the Department of Health and Human Services were hospital cost containment and national health insurance (Stoiber, 1979). Reduction of waste and duplication in the hospital sector was intended to generate the funds for a national health insurance program that would fill the unmet needs for health care. Legislation for national health insurance was considered by Congress but, after much debate, no legislation was adopted and further consideration of national health insurance was dropped. Concern about hospital cost containment continued and was addressed by the Social Security Amendments of 1983, which gave rise to the prospective payment system for Medicare based on diagnosis-related groups.

The second significant trend in the prior decade was rapid change in the relation of health care delivery to the reimbursement for services. Several special issues were raised concerning the new forms of delivery and reimbursement for services, which included health maintenance organizations (HMOs), surgical centers, the expanded role of hospitals for delivery of ambulatory care, hospices, walk-in centers, and multihospital systems. For example, in 1972, legislation was passed to provide grants or loans to support the development of HMOs. Also during the 1970s the federal Administration on Aging began to emphasize that health counseling and health screening should be included in the social services for the elderly provided at the local level under the Older Americans Act. Yet another example was the federal government's response to the shortage of physicians in the 1960s and 1970s. Federal programs for medical students were legislated—programs that stimulated increased enrollments in medical schools and the establishment of new medical services and ultimately resulted in the physician surplus of the 1980s. The full impact of the growing number of physicians on the organization of medical care is not yet clear (Thier, 1986).

Policy is still being driven by financing and organizational questions, but today there is increased emphasis on examining quality-of-care issues, e.g., what health care are the elderly receiving, what good is it doing, and how are the government programs and policies affecting people's lives. This change is a response to issues that have been raised about costs, access to new types of services and technologies, and matching services to the needs of the population generally and, in some instances, to the needs of the elderly specifically.

Implications for the Panel's Approach

The first task of the panel was to make recommendations to improve the data base for health policy for an aging population during the next decade. The panel recognized the difficulties and pitfalls of trying to identify specific policy issues and their related data requirements when looking forward a decade. Such an approach would not only be difficult, but it might also be counterproductive, because policy issues change in unpredictable ways. Accordingly, the panel's recommendations are directed to modifications in the federal statistical system that would ensure the availability of basic data that are relevant and important to the following set of generic health policy issues for an aging society:

- Who will pay for health care for the elderly and how will it be financed?
- What alternative health delivery systems can be developed to meet the needs for health care for the elderly in the next decade?
- How can health promotion and disease prevention be advanced among the elderly?
- How much health care for the elderly will be needed in the next decade? What will the health status of the elderly be in the next decade?

- What are the differences in health status among subgroups of the elderly?
- What policies and programs are needed to ensure that the elderly receive health care of appropriate quality?
- What provisions need to be made for population subgroups to avoid problems of equity and access in health care for the elderly?
- Are health programs and benefits for the elderly equitably distributed across the states? What is the impact of geographic variation?
- Are there unintended effects of government programs for health care for the elderly?

As stated, these health policy issues are sufficiently broad so as to include the specific policy issues of both the past and current decades and can be expected to include those of the next decade.

The special policy issues that arise during a decade are shaped by the trends of the time. In forecasting health policy choices for the 1990s, a variety of demographic, economic, organizational, and attitudinal trends can be expected to shape health policy issues in the 1990s and to change the U.S. health care system (Blendon, 1986). In addition to the growing number of oldest-old, specific trends can be expected to influence policy issues for health care for the elderly, which are detailed below.

The continuing problem of rising health care costs. Despite the continuing efforts to contain them, the nation's health care costs "are projected to increase from $387 billion in 1984 to $660 billion in 1990, reaching almost $2 trillion by 2000" (Blendon, 1986:67). The aging of the population is not the only factor contributing to the rising cost: improved and costly medical technologies and the volume and complexity of new types of services may serve to increase health care costs (Blendon, 1986).

The growing concern with quality of care and cost-benefit ratios, i.e., what government and private purchasers are receiving for their money. Efforts to manage costs and distinguish high-quality care from less effective and less efficient care are stimulating efforts to monitor all sites of care. The monitoring of hospital performance was mandated through provisions of the Social Security Amendments of 1972, requiring that professional standards review organizations (PSROs) be established to ensure that health care services provided under the Medicare and Medicaid programs "were medically necessary, conformed to appropriate professional standards of quality, and were delivered in the most effective and economical manner possible" (National Health Policy Forum, 1985:4). Further changes were made in the TEFRA (Tax Equity and Fiscal Responsibility Act) legislation of 1982, replacing the PSROs with professional review organizations (PROs), which have stronger regulatory powers. In 1986 Congress extended the PRO scope to include review of HMOs and other prepaid plans under contract to provide care to Medicare beneficiaries. The changes also provided for targeted reviews of nursing and home health care services, and (at a later implementation date) services in physicians' offices. As the role of peer review organizations expands, new measures to quantify quality for different services and in different settings will be needed (National Health Policy Forum, 1986).

Continuing rapid change in the organizational structure of the health service delivery system. During the past few years, enrollment of Medicare beneficiaries in HMOS has increased because of federal incentives to HMOs to provide capitated comprehensive care for Medicare patients. In addition, partly in response to the prospective payment system for Medicare inpatient services in hospitals, many new types of out-of-hospital health care facilities have received increased attention. These facilities include ambulatory care centers, diagnostic or imaging centers, hospices, rehabilitation institutes, surgical centers, and urgent care centers. These facilities may be owned by hospitals or hospital chains, for-profit companies, or groups of physicians (Blendon, 1986). Such changes are still evolving and there is no clear indication of the extent to which they will affect the pattern and sources of care for the elderly.

Since it is not possible to predict the effects of these interacting trends and the specific policy issues they may generate, the panel focused on providing a general-purpose statistical base for each of the generic policy issues, keeping in mind the current issues and the foreseeable issues on the horizon. We relied on our knowledge about aging and our experience with data requirements and data gaps in past policy analyses to make determinations about the relevance and importance of data for these generic policy issues.

General-purpose statistics and statistics derived from administrative records for federal programs cannot be expected to supply all the data needed by policy analysts, although the two types of data taken together can answer many questions. For example, the policy question, "Should we be spending more or less on health care for the elderly?" requires information on who is being served and how much is being spent in the aggregate and for which services. Aggregate data from administrative records (e.g., Medicare and Medicaid) can provide information on who is being served and how much is being spent under the programs. The National Medical Expenditure Survey, which surveys a sample of the general population as well as people in institutions, will provide information on expenditures not included in government programs and information on health care expenditures by elderly people who are not participants in these programs. The policy question, "Are the Medicare and Medicaid programs meeting the needs of different categories of the elderly (rural elderly, chronically disabled elderly, etc.), as 'need' is defined by different policy analysts?" calls for evaluations and would probably require special studies, although the national statistics on health service utilization for various subgroups of the population might be the starting point in designing the special study. The policy question, "How much need will there be for health care for the elderly in future years and what will it cost?" may call for a forecast of the quantity of health care that will be needed assuming policy remains unchanged, in which case demographic data, in conjunction with data from the Health Care Financing Administration on Medicare and Medicaid utilization and costs, are essential to answer this question.

Policy analysts frequently require forecasts of the quantity and costs of health care under various hypothetical scenarios, which may have never occurred. A current example of this is found in the eight alternative reform proposals under consideration for redesigning Medicare, which are discussed in a report for the National Health Policy Forum (Etheredge, 1987). One aspect of Medicare benefits under consideration is "Should Medicare eligibility continue to start at age 65, or at younger or older ages?" Forecasts of savings by adopting cutoffs at older ages can be prepared from Medicare data, but the quantity of health services that ended if the eligibility age were changed to 62 (as suggested in one proposal) is more tenuous. The basic data source would be the health service utilization data for ages 62-64 in the National Medical Expenditure Survey. However, since utilization of health services might change under expanded Medicare coverage, data from experience under past policy, although relevant, are not conclusive. In fact, many policy issues cannot be adequately addressed by drawing on general-purpose statistics and data from administrative records. In some cases, a special supplemental survey may be needed. In others, targeted experiments are required to learn about the impact of policy options in many settings.

RECOMMENDATIONS

The multiplicity of agencies concerned with statistics on the elderly and the numerous surveys and administrative record systems involved led the panel to make a large number of recommendations. The organizational structure of the report also contributed to the number of recommendations, since several chapters on different policy areas may have recommendations about a single survey. To guide the reader, we summarize the recommendations in three ways: first, we present a set of 12 specific priority recommendations; second, we present 5 general recommendations that summarize the chapter recommendations; finally, we present a table with the 79 individual recommendations that are discussed in the chapters.

Priority Recommendations

The panel selected these recommendations from the large number of detailed recommendations as those that should be given priority because they will provide the data most urgently needed for health policy for an aging society. The priority recommendations consist of both parts and combinations of recommendations that appear in the chapters. The recommendations are presented in the context of the policy areas they address and are followed by the rationale for each recommendation.

Financing of Medical Care: For the aging population, the major policy issues that will confront the United States during the next decade are the cost of supplying health care to the elderly, who will pay for that care, and how it will be financed.

Policy development for these issues requires trend data on the health expenditures of the elderly and also longitudinal data on the use of medical care as a person ages. In addition, evaluation of policy questions related to the Medicare program would be facilitated by improved access to the Medicare statistical system.

Priority Recommendation 1:   The panel recommends (a) continuation of the periodic survey of national medical care expenditures, the periodicity to be determined in relation to policy needs and timing of other health-related surveys and

(b) that the population age 55 and over in the 1987 survey be identified and followed by linking to administrative records, including Medicare reimbursements from Health Care Financing Administration records, and, to the extent feasible, Medicaid reimbursements from state record systems and work history and pension benefits from Social Security Administration records. In addition, the National Death Index of the National Center for Health Statistics and state health department death records should be used to identify the year and cause of death of each sampled person.

Priority Recommendation 2: The panel recommends that the Health Care Financing Administration develop files designed for easy access to the Medicare Statistical System (including the Medicare Automated Data Retrieval System) that would facilitate use by researchers for policy analysis related to the Medicare program.

Trend data on health expenditures for the elderly. National health expenditure data are widely used by policy makers to evaluate the extent of coverage of existing public programs, such as Medicare and Medicaid, and to estimate the total health care costs of the elderly population by type of expenditure and source of funds. The data also serve as a basis for assessing the possible consequences of changes in public policy programs. The major sources of such data have been the 1980 National Medical Care Utilization and Expenditures Survey (NMCUES) and the 1977 National Medical Care Expenditures Survey (NMCES). These surveys and the Medicare files are the primary data sources for estimating cost and coverage of program changes, such as the various proposals for catastrophic health care coverage currently being considered by Congress. More current data will become available in 1988 from the ongoing 1987 National Medical Expenditure Survey (NMES). The 1980s have been and continue to be a decade of far-reaching changes in the structure of the health care delivery system, private health insurance, federal and state and local health care programs, as well as in the demographic composition of the nation. How these changes affect the kinds and amounts of health care Americans use, how they will pay for it, and the implications of further changes in health care policy are questions that NMES data and the analyses based on them will help to answer.

However, to capture trends in utilization and expenditure patterns in response to future changes in delivery and payment systems over time and to meet policy needs for current data, a survey of national medical care expenditures should be conducted periodically. In order to take full advantage of the various types of relevant expertise in different agencies, future national medical care expenditure surveys should be joint efforts of appropriate federal agencies, including the National Center for Health Services Research and Health Care Technology, the Health Care Financing Administration, and the National Center for Health Statistics.

Longitudinal data for the elderly in NMES through follow-up studies using administrative records. A major gap in understanding the impact of changes in the financing of medical care services for individuals and their families is the lack of longitudinal data on the use of and expenditures for medical care services as a person ages and is at risk of chronic illness requiring acute medical and long-term care services. Since significant changes in health status frequently start to occur in the decade prior to age 65, it is important for longitudinal studies to start following people at age 55.

Extensive additional data about the individuals sampled in the NMES are available from administrative records of the Health Care Financing Administration, the Social Security Administration, and the Internal Revenue Service. Information on the cause of death can be determined through use of the National Death Index maintained by the National Center for Health Statistics and death records in the state health departments. Use of the rich information available from administrative records can enhance the usefulness of survey data collected in the NMES for longitudinal analyses at very low cost.

Improved Access to the Medicare Statistical System. The Medicare Statistical System (MSS) was designed to provide data to measure and evaluate the operation and effectiveness of the Medicare program. It has also been a major source of information for evaluating policy questions relating to the equity and efficiency of the Medicare program. For example, data on the distribution of Medicare reimbursements for survivors and decedents and for type of service provide useful data on the high use and costs of medical care services in the last year of life. Medical reimbursements per capita by state and county are useful measures of equity. Provider certification data related to population are important measures of the supply of facilities and services and their variation across the country. Geographic variations in surgical procedures among the elderly are important indicators of practice patterns. The MSS, a by-product of administrative record systems, includes data on each Medicare enrollee, institutional providers of service, and records of the utilization of services that can be matched to enrollees and providers.

Despite the obvious attractiveness of the Medicare files for analytic purposes, these files were established primarily to assist with administration and monitoring of the Medicare program. To make the Medicare administrative data more accessible and less costly for research use, a new file has been designed—the Medicare Automated Data Retrieval System (MADRS). The MADRS is intended to reorganize and merge claims files for Medicare Part A (hospital insurance) and Part B (supplementary medical insurance for physicians' services, outpatient services, etc.) to shorten search time and will contain all Medicare claims data and patient provider identifiers.

The MADRS file will enable researchers to identify groups of special interest and analyze them by age, by sex, and/or by admitting diagnosis, for example, and examine the care they have received over time. The development of the MADRS is a positive step toward facilitating the analysis of Medicare data, thus gaining a better understanding of trends in health services utilization among the elderly.

The Health Care Financing Administration should develop new approaches to improving access to its administrative files by nonfederal users, such as making arrangements for intergovernmental personnel appointments, interns, and postdoctoral fellows.

Organization and Delivery of Health Services: Cost concerns frequently lead to issues concerning the organization and delivery of health services. Rapid changes are taking place in the health care delivery system; policy makers need to monitor these changes and to assess the effects they are having on health care for the elderly.

Detailed data are needed on changes taking place in the health care delivery system and their effects on health care for the elderly.

Priority Recommendation 3: The panel recommends that federal agencies give high priority to reviewing and modifying the contents of administrative record systems, provider-based surveys, and, to the extent feasible, population-based surveys to reflect the rapidly changing patterns in health service delivery. Standard definitions and formats for recording information on the type of health plan should be used by all agencies collecting such data.

The adoption of the diagnosis-related groups and other prospective payment systems for hospital care, the growth of for-profit health care, the adoption of business-oriented approaches by health care providers, and the growth of competition in the medical care market may cause unintended side-effects, such as barriers to access to health care for certain population subgroups and deterioration in quality of care. The preceding recommendation, if implemented, would provide the data required to monitor the effects of the rapid changes in the health care delivery systems. The modifications recommended should improve the data base for monitoring changes in the organization and delivery of health care service, while adoption of standard definitions will enable interviewers, respondents, and coders to distinguish among the various types of health plans in use, including the varieties of capitated plans; and to detect differences in the cost-sharing provisions of these plans.

Provision for Long-term Care: A major factor in the cost of supplying health care for the elderly is the need for and cost of long-term care. Such care is also the primary concern in many of the issues pertaining to the organization and delivery of care.

The concern about provision of long-term care will lead to policy about its organization, delivery, and financing. Policy makers will need current information about the use of long-term care and data for projecting the need for it as characteristics of the elderly and the nature of their support system changes.

Priority Recommendation 4:   The panel recommends that the National Nursing Home Survey (a) be conducted on a 3-5 year cycle and (b) that a subsample of admission cohorts in the 1985 survey serve as a panel for a longitudinal study of institutionalized persons and that the records of this subsample be linked with Medicare files.

Timely data on long-term care.   The provision of long-term care for the chronically ill and feeble is a major issue related to the aging population. The complex of long-term care issues has surfaced in the current congressional debates on the need for increased Medicare coverage for catastrophic illness, highlighting the need for data on long-term care. Decisions will have to be made, either now or in the near future, about the organization, delivery, and financing of long-term care. The National Nursing Home Survey, conducted by the National Center for Health Statistics in 1973-1974, 1977, and

1985, provides information useful for such decision making. This information includes data on nursing homes, their services, staffs, and financial characteristics, and on the personal and health characteristics of residents and discharges (1985 only). These surveys should be conducted more often than every 6-8 years, however, because of increases in the costs of nursing home care and frequent changes in policy. A 3-year interval, or at most, a 5-year interval, is needed to address issues on changes in health for the elderly, outcomes of care, targeting and substitution of services, and the impact of policy changes.

Data for projecting the need for long-term care. By definition, long-term care is care over an extended time period. To project the need for long-term care, data are required for a relatively long period on changes in the characteristics of the elderly population, their use of services, and the nature of their support system, as well as changes in this system, both formal and informal. The 1977 and 1985 National Nursing Home Surveys are useful models for longitudinal surveys of the institutionalized elderly. The 1985 survey included a follow-up of discharged patients. Data were collected from next of kin of both residents and discharged patients on functional disability at time of admission, caregiver stress, and the family's view of the reasons for admission. Surveys of this type conducted at relatively frequent intervals with longitudinal follow-up as recommended above would provide much of the data required for policy decisions on long-term care.

Over time, the National Nursing Home Survey should be expanded to include all types of long-term care institutions (i.e., chronic disease hospitals, mental health facilities, rehabilitation centers, board and care homes, psychiatric halfway houses, and residential facilities. Expanding the coverage of the survey in this manner would make it possible to compare the costs of other modes of providing long-term care services, costs that are essential to planning the organization and delivery of long-term care services. The National Center for Health Statistics took the first step in expanding coverage with the 1980-1981 development efforts to expand the coverage of the Master Facilities List. It would also be desirable to link the records of the longitudinal subsample with Medicaid records, since Medicaid is a major source of support for nursing home care. At present, however, there are problems in linking into Medicaid information on a national scale.

Health Promotion and Disease Prevention in the Elderly: A wise

investment strategy would support spending health care dollars to lengthen the period of life spent in vigorous health. Expenditures for health promotion may well lead to more years of good health than equal expenditures on medical care directed to treating disabilities and serious or irreversible disease. Related policy issues include how health promotion activities can be advanced among the elderly, whether the federal government should fund health promotion and disease prevention activities, and, if so, which ones.

The paucity of data concerning health promotion and disease prevention activities among the elderly creates barriers to the development of policies that recognize this aspect of health care.

Priority Recommendation 5: The panel recommends (a) that modules of health promotion and disease prevention items (including those concerned with attitudes, knowledge, and behavior) be developed that are appropriate for the elderly and subgroups of the elderly population at risk for particular diseases, illnesses, disabilities, or conditions, which can be used with a variety of population-based surveys; (b) that these modules be tested on relevant segments of the elderly population; and (c) that successful modules be incorporated in population-based surveys such as the National Health Interview Survey and the National Health and Nutrition Examination Survey, or as supplements to them.

Health promotion and disease prevention are a major emerging theme in geriatric medicine and health care generally. Although such efforts have typically been targeted at younger persons, there is growing evidence that this approach is both appropriate and feasible for persons 65 and over. Health promotion and disease prevention are one of a number of possible strategies to deal with the prevalence of chronic illness and multiple chronic illnesses or functional impairments among the elderly. While this approach will neither replace medical care for the treatment of acute diseases, nor for acute flare-ups of chronic illness, it has promise for reducing or delaying the incidence and prevalence of chronic and acute disease among both the general population and the elderly.

Despite the obvious importance of health promotion and disease prevention, data are not routinely available through national data systems on the extent to which the population is informed as to the causes of preventable illnesses and conditions and the actions they might take to reduce their own risks of developing such illnesses and accompanying impairments. Development of the recommended modules will require cooperation and coordination of effort by several agencies, including the Office of Health Promotion and Disease Prevention, the National Center for Health Services Research and Health Care Technology, and institutes within the National Institutes of Health.

Monitoring and Forecasting Health Status and the Utilization of Services: Assessment of the cost of supplying health care to the elderly will require estimates of the health care needs of the elderly, what types of care will be needed, and to what extent needs are met. This requires periodic monitoring of the health status of the elderly and their use of health care services to detect trends and to forecast future health status and utilization of services.

The information needed for such monitoring and forecasting includes longitudinal data on aging and information on the relation between health status and health services utilization. In addition, an evaluation of the theory, methodology, and data requirements for forecasting the characteristics of the aging population is needed.

Priority Recommendation 6: The panel recommends that the National Center for Health Statistics (a) continue to collect, every two years, health and other relevant information (hospital and physician care, income, housing, informal support, and the use of community services) from all persons age 55 and older in the original sample of persons in the 1984 Supplement on Aging of the National Health Interview Survey, now known as the Longitudinal Study on Aging, (b) use the National Health Interview Survey as a base for a periodic Supplement on Aging for the noninstitutionalized population age 55 and over, and (c) conduct follow-up interviews of the supplemental sample to provide longitudinal as well as cross-sectional data on the older population.

Priority Recommendation 7: The panel recommends that (a) linkage with Medicare records be performed on a routine basis for persons age 65 and over who are respondents to population surveys that collect health data and (b) the Health Care Financing Administration and the National Center for Health Statistics explore linking the Health Interview Survey with the Medicare Automated Data Retrieval System, when the latter becomes operational.

Priority Recommendation 8:   The panel recommends that a study to evaluate theoretical, methodological, and data requirements for forecasting the characteristics of the aging population be undertaken. This would include theoretical and practical considerations for evaluating the sensitivity of forecasts to underlying assumptions.

Longitudinal data on aging.   Many questions concerning the health and functional status of the elderly remain unanswered at this time. In particular, the dynamic process of how individuals change in health and functional status as they grow older, and the nature of the critical transitions they experience as they pass from one health or functional status to another, are not well understood. This information is basic in determining whether and how various subgroups of the elderly population are changing in their patterns of morbidity, functioning, and quality of life, information essential for determination of future health care needs and expenditures as longevity of the population increases. Repeated measures of the same individual over time are needed to elucidate these processes and changes and provide information for health policy making.

A promising medium for obtaining such information is the 1984 Supplement on Aging (SOA) of the National Health Interview Survey. This supplement collected data on a sample of 8,000 persons age 55 and over in the community. In addition to information on health status and hospital and physician care, this survey collected information on income, housing, informal support, and the use of social services. Persons age 70 and over in 1974 were reinterviewed in 1986. Additional reinterviewing of this sample and periodic repetition of the SOA with longitudinal follow-ups would permit measurement of some of the transitions occurring in the elderly population. The follow-up could be carried out by a combination of telephone calls and personal interviews with varying frequencies appropriate to the age of the sample member. Rapid changes in health, medical care needs, living arrangements, and available support are characteristic of the older population and must be understood to forecast the health services needs of the future elderly.

Relationship between health status and health services utilization. It is important to be able to relate the health and personal status of the elderly to their utilization of health services so that trends in health status can be used to forecast patterns of change in health service utilization. Many population surveys, including the National Health Interview Survey, the National Medical Expenditure Survey, the National Nursing Home Survey, and the Survey on Income and Program Participation, obtain important demographic and health status information that can be linked with Medicare file data for the same individuals. Such linkages could provide a rich source of longitudinal information on health services utilization by the elderly, making it possible to relate health status and other characteristics to subsequent use of health services.

Forecasts of the characteristics of the aging population. Many of the factors that are of interest for an aging population interact with one another. One way to account for such interactions is through global models that attempt to integrate different submodels or modules into a common projection framework. Integrated efforts are necessary to forecast health status, functional limitations, and support systems available for older persons. These forecasts can be useful not only for probing important policy issues related to health care expenditures and welfare programs, but also for improved mortality forecasts in general population projections.

Ensuring That Health Care Meets Quality Standards: **Questions about the quality of care are an integral part of the debate on cost containment policies for health care for the elderly and the consequences of adopted policies. Policy makers will require indicators on quality of care to inform this debate.**

A concerted effort is needed to develop measures of quality of care of elderly patients that are suitable for national data systems.

> **Priority Recommendation 9:** The panel recommends that agencies having cognizance of national data systems, whether based on administrative records or survey data, (a) jointly review these data systems to identify items that can be used in developing quality of care measures and to identify missing items that are needed to produce such measures and (b) make provision for collecting the needed data and for producing quality of care measures.

Quality of care is emerging as a matter of central interest for policies directed at controlling costs or improving services for specific subgroups of the elderly. An Office of Technology Assessment report to Congress (Office of Technology Assessment, 1985a) pointed out that assessing the effects of Medicare's prospective payment system on quality of care is critical. The Institute of Medicine's recent report on quality of care in nursing homes (Institute of Medicine,

1986) identifies the need for a system of acquiring and using resident assessment data.

The context for quality of care issues will broaden as policies to control costs are extended to sectors other than hospital care and as alternative sources of care become available, particularly for long-term care patients.

National data systems can produce the information needed to derive quality of care measures to determine how quality varies within the population and how it may be influenced by sources of care and policies that affect services received. Many of the specific items required are included in surveys that are already operational or about to start; others are dependent on the extension of existing items or the introduction of new ones. Candidates are found in the National Health Interview Survey and its supplements on aging and prevention, the National Nursing Home Survey, the National Health and Nutrition Examination Survey, the National Ambulatory Medical Care Survey (NCHS), the Long-Term Care Survey (HCFA), and in the forthcoming National Medical Expenditures Survey (NCHSR and HCFA).

Not only should national data systems be able to measure quality directly, but they should also provide broad indicators of quality of care that will alert policy makers that other information is needed. For example, in 1986, when the Health Care Financing Administration released mortality data (an outcome measure for quality of care) for 2,300 hospitals and identified 269 institutions in which death rates were significantly higher or lower than others, the response was to focus attention on how patients are managed in hospitals. The hospital industry argued that the data were misleading because they did not take into consideration factors such as severity of illness or the extent to which high-risk procedures are performed in specialty hospitals. This led to increased efforts to develop measures of severity of illness (Horn and Horn, 1986).

The panel considers the development of measures of quality of care of elderly patients that are suitable for national data systems to be a high-priority effort. At the same time, we recognize the inherent difficulties because there is no accepted definition of quality of care and because of the conceptual problem of quantifying good quality.

Improving the Quality of Health Policy Analysis: Procedural recommendations to improve access to data or the capability to analyze data from multiple sources cut across policy issues. Increased detail in publication of data, improved access to data, and planning and coordination of data collections to provide the capability of inter-relating the data from different sources can improve the quality of policy analysis and extend the scope of policy-oriented research.

The panel makes three recommendations on these activities.

Priority Recommendation 10: The panel recommends that agencies that collect and disseminate data on the total population or administrative data by age (a) use 5-year age groups for the publication of data up to age 90 and larger intervals thereafter, except when limited by privacy or confidentiality regulations and (b) provide data on geographic areas, income, and other economic characteristics at the greatest level of detail consistent with the protection of confidentiality.

Priority Recommendation 11: The panel recommends that the plans of a federal agency for the creation or continuation of a data system include a plan for issuance of publications and public use tapes following its creation or updating. The plan should include explicit procedures for disseminating the data and should provide for widespread access and timely, thorough, and accurate data dissemination.

Priority Recommendation 12: The panel recommends that a mechanism be provided for discussion and coordination of data needs, standardized definitions and classifications, priority identification, and production of data relating to an aging society.

Data detail. As the elderly population increases in size and as a proportion of the total population, it becomes increasingly important to know more about specific groups within that population. For different purposes, additional detail may be needed on the oldest-old, five-year age groups among the elderly, women, minorities, persons with health problems, the poor elderly, and other special populations. Frequently information issued in aggregate form does not include enough detail to identify these subpopulations. For data from administrative records or from the decennial census, the failure to meet these needs of policy analysts is a matter of presentation. The single most useful standard that agencies could adopt is to provide information for standard age categories in publications and public use files.

Improved access to data. To make data more accessible to researchers and to increase the usefulness of data for policy purposes, tape files for research use need to be created in federal statistical and administrative programs without violating confidentiality. The agencies should also conduct more outreach programs to inform potential users of the availability of tapes and provide training on their use. For example, the National Center for Health Statistics has a program for informing potential users of the availability of data tapes and how to use them; a series of "Advance Data" releases are also distributed before final figures are available.

Planning and coordination of data collections. In a decentralized federal data system, such as exists in the United States, it is especially important to have some mechanism for planning and coordinating the disparate activities of different federal agencies that are engaged in collecting information about the elderly. The purpose of the newly established Forum on Aging-Related Statistics, which includes representatives from all the federal agencies that collect statistical information on the elderly, is to encourage cooperation among these agencies in the development, collection, analysis, and dissemination of data on the older population.

General Recommendations

The preceding priority recommendations come from a substantially larger set of specific recommendations that reflect the full range of the panel's findings and conclusions. The detailed recommendations are intended to provide the basis for making current data collection efforts more effective and for providing necessary supplements to those efforts. Table 1.1 at the end of this chapter lists short titles of *all* the recommendations given in each chapter with the agencies whose involvement would be required to implement each recommendation. The priority recommendations discussed above are indicated by a P in the table. Recommendations that entail conducting surveys appear in the table under the appropriate statistical agency(ies), but not under research sponsoring agencies that might provide support for the surveys. The panel recognizes that such support is essential for near-term implementation of some recommendations, particularly those assigned a priority.

In this section, five general recommendations provide an integrated picture of the full set of recommendations. They represent the collection and integration of a number of specific recommendations that follow in subsequent chapters.

- **Develop and maintain a core group of national longitudinal health surveys to study health transitions and health service needs among the elderly.**

Nationally representative longitudinal data are needed to accurately describe the health and functional transitions of the old and oldest-old U.S. populations. Purely cross-sectional data may provide erroneous and incomplete insights to these processes and miss important underlying changes. To develop accurate nationally representative data on the health and functional changes of the elderly, and the relation of those changes to recent life expectancy changes, existing national surveys of the major population groups of the elderly need to be supplemented by longitudinal follow-up of selected survey cohorts. And these reinterview programs need to be supplemented by the linkage of the survey records to Medicare Part A and B data files and to death certificates identified through the National Death Index.

The minimal core of longitudinal surveys for adequate population coverage are the survey programs that produced the 1984 Health Interview Survey, the Supplement on Aging (SOA) and the 1986 follow-up Longitudinal Study on Aging (LSOA), the 1985 National Nursing Home Survey (NNHS) and the 1987 follow-up, and the 1982 and 1984 National Long-Term Care Surveys (NLTCS), and the follow-up studies of the National Health and Nutrition Examination Survey (NHANES) populations. The first three of these surveys cover the major elderly population components (i.e., the SOA-LSOA, the general elderly population; the NNHS, the institutionalized population; the NLTCS, the community-disabled elderly). The fourth, the NHANES with expanded follow-up studies, would provide longitudinal biomedical and epidemiological information. Although these four surveys provide an excellent basis for a national set of longitudinal surveys, they have been hampered in design and coverage by inadequate and unstable funding. More adequate levels of funding could make these surveys more effective by:

- ensuring follow-ups at regular periods,
- improving instrument design and measurement,
- ensuring cross-sectional representativeness of the total U.S. elderly population by enrolling samples of the population that become elderly between survey dates,

- making the sample design more effective by conducting more intensive sampling of special target populations (e.g., over-sampling the population age 85 and older in future supplements on aging in the Health Interview Survey),
- providing for assessment of short-term changes by more frequent follow-ups of sample subpopulations.

- **Introduce design changes in other major survey programs to improve their usefulness for studying the health of the elderly, health care expenditures, and quality of care.**

A number of existing major surveys such as the National Medical Expenditure Survey (on the health expenditures of the general U.S. population), the National Ambulatory Medical Care Survey (NAMCS) (on the use of office-based physician services, health problems, and diagnostic and therapeutic services received by the general U.S. population), and the Survey of Income and Program Participation (SIPP) (on the income, assets, and program participation of both young and old Americans), provide valuable information on a series of special topics. Furthermore, certain surveys like the NHIS, the NNHS and the NMES represent long-term and continuous survey efforts. Thus these surveys merit continuing support—both because of the information they currently generate and because of the increased value of that information in the context of a long time series of such surveys, extending from 1957 in the case of the NHIS, 1963 in the case of the NNHS, and 1977 in the case of the NMES.

Changes have been made in these surveys recently and additional changes are needed. Though crucial to continue, these surveys must be carefully assessed for needed changes in the measurement, survey, and sample design to improve their effectiveness. Specific examples of possible needed changes are: (a) increased oversampling of the old and oldest-old in the NMES and the SIPP, (b) repeating the health module at least twice in the SIPP survey cycle, (c) improving the quality of care measures in the NHIS, and (d) developing and introducing health promotion and disease prevention items in the NHIS, the NHANES, or supplements to them, and the NAMCS. In general the adequacy of sample sizes for special subpopulations (such as the 85 years and older population) should be evaluated in all such surveys, and their periodicity and the quality of their health instruments need to be assessed.

Before such changes could be introduced two types of research will be needed. The first is evaluation studies of the current content, sample design, periodicity, population coverage, and overlap of these surveys. Such studies will require special and adequate funding to the appropriate technical groups within the National Center for Health Statistics and the Census Bureau. The results of such studies must be reviewed for technical merit by an independent group before instituting changes to ensure that (a) changes will improve the technical quality of the effort and (b) the substantive continuity of the existing time series will be maintained. Part of this evaluation process should involve assessment by the appropriate agencies of whether the necessary data are being collected to serve national health policy needs, to monitor the health of the nation, and for scientific purposes. For example, in terms of meeting public health and scientific needs, such surveys should be reviewed by technical groups appointed by the federal Forum on Aging-Related Statistics, which involves the Census Bureau, the National Center for Health Statistics, the National Institute on Aging, and other agencies.

The second type of studies is scientific investigations of data collection methodologies (e.g., studies of instrumentation, sample design, and periodicity). The studies should be supported through the appropriate extramural research programs at the National Institute on Aging and the National Science Foundation using supplementary funding identified specifically for these purposes.

- **Standardize definitions and instrumentation across data collection and data dissemination activities.**

A number of efforts should be made to ensure comparability between different data collection and dissemination efforts. For example, a standard definition of long-term care should be adopted. To give another example, in disseminating population data adequate age detail is necessary (e.g., by five-year age groups to age 90 and larger intervals thereafter). By establishing standard categories with adequate detail in published documents the utility of multiple data collection efforts will be enhanced.

There is much to be gained from the standardization of certain basic content modules to facilitate comparability across surveys. For example, basic income and assets questions might be standardized, as might certain basic instrumentation for functional assessment, for health promotion and disease prevention activities, and for measuring quality of care. The efforts of interagency committees to generate such standardization should be facilitated by appropriate levels of support.

- **Improve mechanisms for the broad dissemination of all types of data collected with federal support.**

With both the existing and proposed federal data collection efforts, there should be rapid and broad circulation of data generated from all types of federally supported research and data collection. That is, part of our current inability to respond to certain major policy and scientific questions is that data already collected are not available until several years after collection. Federal policy should mandate that all federally funded survey efforts be made publicly available as soon as possible. Included in such releases should also be all linked information, e.g., linked Medicare service use records. Federal data policies must be changed to make such provisions.

- **Provide an adequate level of support for statistical and forecasting research.**

Federal data collection efforts, to be maximally effective, must be supported by appropriate methodological research on the analysis of longitudinal data from repeated cross-sectional and longitudinal surveys. Such methodological research should incorporate research on design of data collection such as the dimensions of measurement, survey design, sample design, linkage to continuous longitudinal administrative records, the issue of the correct temporal spacing of repeated surveys, treatment of missing data in longitudinal studies, and the calculation of power for multivariate cross-temporal data. Analytic research issues center around retrieving estimates of parameters from process models of health and functional changes at advanced ages from incompletely observed processes. In addition, research is needed on how multiple surveys can be integrated in coordinated analyses and on the use of such data in forecasting. There is also a need for research on the forecasting of health, disability, and mortality in the U.S. elderly and oldest-old populations. The research should examine such questions as how to represent the effects of social and economic changes on health transitions, how to determine the uncertainty of forecasts, and how new data will affect the degree of uncertainty. Such methodological research should be supported by extramural research programs at the National Science Foundation and the National Institute on Aging.

A Word About Costs

When grouped according to their expected costs, the panel's recommendations consist of 4 groups: (1) recommendations that fall within the scope of routine operations, either administrative or research and development, and could be implemented within the current staffing configurations of the relevant agency; (2) recommendations that require special studies, analyses, or projections; (3) recommendations for research to develop additional survey methodology or methodology for statistical and policy analysis; and (4) recommendations to augment the scope or content of data sources, to increase the periodicity of surveys, to follow samples of existing surveys to obtain longitudinal data, and to increase survey sample size to provide age detail for the elderly.

Half the recommendations fall in the first group, and although these recommendations are not cost-free, they do not entail additional costs. A fifth of the recommendations fall in the second and third groups and require special studies or research projects that would probably cost between $200,000 and $300,000 (in 1987 dollars) each. For many of the 25 recommendations in the fourth group, the associated costs may exceed $500,000 each. It is important to remember that the costs would be spread over the 21 agencies to which recommendations are addressed as well as the breadth of efforts covered and the range and importance of issues to which these data can be applied.

The panel discussed the feasibility of estimating the financial and staff resources that would be required to implement this fourth group of recommendations. However, there are several arguments against estimating resource requirements. The panel's recommendations were intended for implementation over the next decade as they fit into agency plans, and estimates made today could be unrealistic in the future and might even be a barrier to implementation. The panel might have requested the federal agencies designated to implement the recommendations to make cost estimates, but it is unlikely that they would be willing to do so unless plans for the recommended activity were currently under discussion. On the basis of these arguments, and since our charge did not call for cost estimates, the panel decided against making estimates of the funds required to implement the recommendations in group 4. In any event, the supplemental funds required to implement the panel's recommendations are minuscule compared with the amount of money expended on major federal and state health programs—far less than would be reasonable for the combined purposes of policy development, program management, evaluation, and research for a major public enterprise.

It is logical to ask whether the benefits that would accrue from implementing these recommendations warrant the cost. Some of the benefits are obvious. The information that would be produced would enhance policy makers' ability to target health care to those in need, increase equity in the allocation of Medicaid funds, control the escalating costs of Medicare, and identify alternative forms of long-term care that might provide cost savings or increased quality of life for the elderly. Since it is particularly difficult to place dollar values on quality of life and access to health care, it was not feasible for the panel to quantify this type of benefit. Therefore, we assigned priority to recommendations that respond to the most pressing needs for information to meet the overall goals of medical care for the elderly. These goals include the following: to enable the elderly to stay healthy and functionally independent as long as possible, to provide access to good medical care of whatever type is appropriate (preventive, long-term, short-term, acute), and to provide care in the least restrictive and most cost-effective and appropriate environment (Somers, 1987).

ORGANIZATION OF THE REPORT

Structure of the Report

The panel's three charges are addressed in separate chapters of the report. Chapter 2 summarizes the social, economic, and demographic trends that trigger policy issues in several topics related to the health of the elderly. Chapters 3-9 discuss the data requirements for policy development for health care for the elderly during the next decade and recommend actions needed to ensure that these data will be available. These chapters correspond to the topic "health policy issues for the elderly" discussed earlier in this chapter. Chapter 10 addresses statistical problems that cut across the federal statistical system. Chapter 11 discusses methodological issues common to many of the data collection efforts and to the use of the data in policy analysis. We summarize the chapter contents below.

Chapter 2: Social, Economic, and Demographic Changes Among the Elderly

Not only is the population aging, but also other major life-course changes are occurring. Age-related roles are less predictable than they were in the past. Late adulthood has a perplexing number of possible life patterns. Trends that should be taken into account in policy analysis on aging include demographic trends, morbidity and mortality patterns, changes in family structure, an increase in the interruption of marital careers, increased mobility, changes in living arrangements, labor force participation, and other activity patterns of the elderly.

The magnitudes of these changes and the acceleration of some of them underscore the importance of well-designed statistical programs to monitor the characteristics of the aging population. The trends and projections based on the trends not only influence program size, but also, in some cases, may influence policy.

Chapters 3 and 4: Health Status, Quality of Life, and Health Transitions

In order to develop policy for health care for the elderly, information is required on trends in health status and utilization of health care to be able to make projections. While there is no doubt that life expectancy is on the rise, a major unanswered question is whether increased longevity will be accompanied by vitality and "active life expectancy," or rather by a prolongation of the period of morbidity and disability and corresponding increments in health services utilization and health care expenditures. Will the added years of life be spent in wellness and the enjoyment of high quality of life, or in relative deprivation due to the presence of irremediable chronic ailments and functional impairments? Chapters 3 and 4 review the data series available for monitoring health status, quality of life, and health transitions and make recommendations to fill serious data gaps.

Chapter 5: Health Promotion and Disease Prevention

In this chapter health promotion and disease prevention are defined and their relevance and the appropriateness of this approach for the elderly are discussed. The chapter explores the need for data concerning the extent to which the elderly are knowledgeable about and engage in health promotion and disease prevention activities and the services in these areas provided to the elderly by health care personnel and institutional providers.

Chapter 6: Quality of Care

A major concern in health care is the quality of care. Policies directed at controlling costs, such as hospital diagnostic-related groups, or at improving services for specific groups of the population, such as the elderly, have made this a matter of immediate interest. In assessing the quality of care provided, not only is the technical performance of health care providers at issue, but also the extent to which the health care system reaches those in need. This chapter underscores the importance of developing indicators of quality of care.

Chapter 7: Long-term Care

The purposes of long-term care services are to assist persons who have lost some capacity for self-care to cope with their disabilities, to decrease their dependence on others, and to narrow the gap between their actual and potential functioning. This chapter reviews the capacity of national data systems to track users of long-term care services over time and to measure and report the services they use.

Chapters 8 and 9: Financing and Utilization of Health Care Services

Chapter 8 describes current mechanisms for financing health care services for the elderly, including the federal Medicare and state Medicaid programs, Veterans Administration services, and private health insurance programs. Health care expenditures for the elderly are also summarized. The chapter explores the potential for extracting more timely and comprehensive financing and expenditure data from the Medicare Statistical System and from planned and existing national health surveys. Particular attention is paid to data that can be used to document the impact of recent changes in health care delivery systems and financing mechanisms, and the effects of the "spend-down" phenomenon on family members.

Chapter 9 reviews the many factors in addition to need that influence the amount and types of health care services utilized by older persons. The focus is on improvements in national data, particularly in the areas of changing service delivery patterns, dental care, rehabilitative care, mental health services, and access to care on the part of poor and other special populations such as the rural elderly.

Chapter 10: Enhancing the Usefulness of National Statistical Systems

Attention is drawn to the need for the federal government to provide greater interagency coordination, cooperation, and planning among those federal agencies and programs that produce statistics on the elderly. Since the United States has a decentralized statistical system, special efforts are required to ensure that data policies across federal agencies and programs are consistent. Coordination of statistics on the elderly is needed with respect to content; coverage; age detail; definitions, concepts, and classification; periodicity; and access to data. The chapter also argues for increased use of linkage among data sets as a mechanism to enhance information about the elderly and suggests ways to improve the vital statistics program and data on causes of death. Furthermore, health-related policy, like other domains of public policy in recent years, is jointly planned and carried out at state and local levels (e.g., Medicaid and the Older Americans Act); consequently the chapter also considers the importance of the collection and timely dissemination of subnational data.

Chapter 11: Methodological and Statistical Issues

The final chapter discusses methodological and statistical issues relevant to an aging society under four headings: the design and analysis of longitudinal studies, linkage of data bases, forecasting the characteristics of future elderly cohorts, and the quantification of uncertainty of projections.

Projecting and Determining Statistical Needs

Several considerations cut across the data requirements for health policy issues addressed in subsequent chapters of the report and provide a unifying framework for the report. These considerations include the need for information on the healthy as well as the dependent elderly, data on functioning to supplement diagnostic information, longitudinal data on the elderly, information on the responsiveness of the elderly to both acute and long-term care systems, better information about long-term care services provided to the elderly, data on risk factors for the elderly, better data on special subgroups of the elderly, and forecasts of the characteristics of future cohorts of elderly.

Information on the Healthy Elderly

Contrary to popular belief or stereotype, the elderly are highly diverse with respect to just about any characteristic, whether it be health or functional status, economic or social circumstances, or living arrangements. Frailty, ill health, and disability increase, on the average, with age, and data on this process are needed. But many elderly persons are in excellent health and function independently in most if not all areas of their lives. These persons often experience a high quality of life and engage in satisfying productive activity, underscoring the need to focus greater attention in data collection efforts on the well and independent elderly. The level of dependence of the elderly in activities of daily living, their physical and/or mental impairments, and their illnesses and disabilities have been the focus of many studies or surveys. Collecting more information on the well and independent elderly will contribute to a better understanding of the factors that lead to positive health and the conditions under which the elderly are able to cope effectively with advancing age.

Data on Functioning to Supplement Diagnostic Information

While health status and the presence or absence of illness and disease are major sources of satisfaction or dissatisfaction with life for older persons, it is the ability to function independently—physically, cognitively, emotionally, and socially—that is crucial to a feeling of well-being and a high quality of life. Diagnostic information is therefore important, as is increased understanding of the effect of different conditions on functional status. However, specific diagnoses often bear no relation to the ability to function nor to the needs and capabilities of an elderly person. New measures of functional status and their incorporation into surveys involving the elderly are needed.

Longitudinal Data on the Elderly

There is a dearth of information about what happens to the elderly as they age—how their health, functional status, economic status, living arrangements, need for long-term care, and utilization of health services interact and change. There is now considerable evidence that there is plasticity in the aging process—that disease processes can be significantly altered or reversed with appropriate therapies. Improvements in health and function over time, as well as decrements, need to be determined for the elderly population. Only repeated measurements of these phenomena over time as a person gets older will yield information on the transitions in health status that occur and circumstances that influence these transitions.

Information on the Responsiveness of Both Acute and Long-term Care Systems

Too often the public equates geriatric medicine with long-term or chronic care. A substantial portion of the health care utilization and expenditures of the elderly, however, is for acute care provided by short-stay hospitals or in the physician's office. The elderly are likely to need both acute and long-term care services at different points in their lives. Because of the many changes in the health care delivery system, in the costs and financing of health care services for the elderly, and in the types and qualifications of health care providers available to them, it is especially important to monitor and document the impact of these changes on the types, amounts, and quality of acute and long-term care services utilized by the elderly. With the introduction of prospective payment systems, based on hospital diagnosis-related groups, there is some evidence that elderly persons are being discharged from acute care facilities sooner than was the case previously, and thus there is the strong possibility that long-term care facilities are receiving more acutely ill persons than they did in the past. Furthermore, the acute care needs of the elderly are different from those of younger persons, and improved data regarding the use and costs of acute and long-term care services by the elderly could assist health care facilities and providers in planning for increased demands on them from the growing elderly population.

Better Information About Long-term Care Services

Long-term health care refers to the professional or personal services required on a recurring or continuous basis by an individual because of chronic or permanent physical or mental impairment.

There is considerable diversity in the types of long-term care services used by the elderly, the settings in which they are provided, the costs of such care to the elderly and their families, and how costs are met. These services may range from informal supports provided by family or friends in the person's home, to paid medical and related social services provided on a periodic or routine basis in the home, to community-based adult day care programs, to custodial, intermediate, or skilled care provided in residential facilities. Because the elderly are the population group most likely to need long-term care, it is important that surveys—and particularly longitudinal surveys—provide more complete information concerning the changes they experience in their use of different levels of care. Such information would provide data needed in planning how to reduce the financial impact of long-term care and make the financing of insurance coverage for institutional care, in particular, feasible.

Data on Risk Factors for the Elderly

Variables identified as risk factors for disease among middle-aged persons, i.e., for the development of stroke, cancer, and heart disease, often differ for persons age 65 and over. Many questions are being raised about how applicable the knowledge developed from studies of persons in their young and middle years is for the elderly. Risk factors at advanced ages have not been adequately studied. The importance of these questions increases as the elderly become more numerous and the proportion at the most advanced ages grows. Better data are needed to identify the specific geriatric syndromes that predispose the elderly to frailty and to establish the risk factors for particular diseases, as well as the risk for developing functional impairment.

Better Data on Special Subgroups of the Elderly

The elderly population that is age 85 and over, the oldest-old, is growing very rapidly both in absolute numbers and as a percentage of the population over age 65; it is expected to grow even more rapidly in the next several decades. Whereas between 1950 and 1980 the population age 65 and over more than doubled, the subpopulation age 85 and over quadrupled in that period, increasing in number from 577,000 in 1950 to 2.2 million in 1980. Inadequate provision has been made for developing information through national surveys for various subgroups of the elderly population.

Blacks, Hispanics, and the poor and near-poor are likely to differ from the remainder of the elderly population in health status and other characteristics. These subgroups should be carefully monitored, and oversampled in surveys if need be, for their health status and health-related service utilization because of their particular vulnerability and potential difficulties in obtaining access to care.

The veteran population, mainly men, is of interest because of the current rapid increase in the number who are elderly. In 1980 there were 3 million veterans age 65 and over, constituting 10.5 percent of the veteran population. It is estimated that by 1990 there will be 7.2 million veterans age 65 and over, constituting 26.6 percent of the veteran population. By 2000, there will be some 9 million veterans age 65 and over, and by 2020 the veteran population age 65 and over will grow to about 45 percent of all veterans. (Veterans Administration, 1984:4). In 1980, 27 percent of all American males age 65 and over were veterans, while in 2000, some 63 percent of American males of that age group will be veterans.

In the veteran population, as in the general population, especially large increases are occurring among those age 75-84 and 85 and older. These subgroups consume the greatest amount of health resources on a per capita basis. Accordingly, the Veterans Administration will face the problems of increased health needs and costs. The data needs identified in this report for the elderly population are relevant for the Veterans Administration, modified by special conditions such as benefit entitlement provisions and availability of health care resources.

Characteristics of Future Cohorts of Elderly

Public policy makers need disaggregated projections of the characteristics of future cohorts of elderly persons—their size; age, sex, race, and ethnic composition; marital status; morbidity and mortality rates; educational and economic status; labor force participation; and housing and living arrangements. Successive cohorts of elderly will differ from each other in these and other respects. Planning for the types and modes of delivery of health care and related services to be provided, how they will be paid and financed, and the numbers of institutional and professional health care providers required to meet the needs of the elderly in future years are heavily dependent on accurate projections of the characteristics of future generations of elderly.

Important Data Bases Outside the Scope of the Report

This report addresses data requirements that can be met by federal agencies responsible for producing policy-relevant information on the state of health of the elderly population, their use of health care resources for acute and long-term conditions, and government and private expenditures for their health care. The information may come from administrative records, statistical surveys, or the decennial census.

The strength and significance of the information systems developed by federal agencies derive largely from the fact that they are national in coverage and produce data on a continuous or periodic basis for demographic, social, and economic subgroups of the population. These systems have been and will continue to be the main source of data needed to understand the current status and trends in health affairs. The recent increased emphasis on longitudinal data has added a new dimension to their potential for answering questions about our aging society's health needs.

Although these systems are an essential source of data for health policy makers, public and private planners, and administrators, there are limits to the scope and detail of the information on the elderly such systems can be expected to provide. Our comprehension of many aspects of health among the elderly is extended beyond what can be gained from multipurpose national data systems by research projects funded by grants or contracts.

The panel is cognizant of the breadth of research on the elderly funded by the National Institute on Aging (NIA), the National Institute of Mental Health (NIMH), the National Center for Health Services Research and Health Care Technology Assessment (NCHSR), and other government agencies and foundations. The symbiotic relationship that exists between these sources and the national data systems has paid dividends and needs to be preserved. In fact, many of the recommendations from the panel regarding data gaps, the need for longitudinal studies, and improved methodologies are relevant for both types of data sources, despite their differences.

National systems can identify major characteristics of health-related problems and progress in dealing with them. Research projects can probe more intensively into selected issues and influence the national systems. Research is often directed at specific health conditions, their incidence and prevalence, associated functional impairment, and factors affecting amelioration or deterioration. Etiological questions and some issues of transition may best be dealt with through research projects that utilize local cohorts monitored carefully at frequent intervals. Many investigations are theoretically based and are designed to test hypotheses; others break open new fields of inquiry through advances in methodology and instrument development.

A detailed discussion of specific projects is beyond the scope of this report, but a few examples illustrate their significance. The Epidemiologic Catchment Area (ECA) research program, conducted cooperatively between NIMH and academically based investigators in five local areas of the country, is the source for the most extensive data on the epidemiology of mental health disorders and related health services available in the United States. Oversampling of the elderly in the surveys carried out has made it possible to give them major attention. Prospects for periodic reexamination of mental disorders are increased through transfer of portions of the Diagnostic Interview Schedule in the ECA to national surveys.

The surveys called Established Populations for Epidemiologic Studies of the Elderly (EPESE) are sponsored by NIA under contract in four areas. New knowledge is being developed concerning medical and social factors in health conditions among the elderly (e.g., pain, sleep, hearing, vision) through annual, intensive surveys of panels of subjects. The Durham Older Americans Resources and Services (OARS) Community Survey at Duke University has conducted locally based longitudinal studies of older people and has adapted and tested instruments for measuring their functional status.

To these can be added other highly targeted studies supported by agencies inside and outside government. An important development in more recent years to increase the utility of data collection in research projects has been the establishment of archives of information for secondary data analysis by scholars here and abroad. An example of this is the National Archive of Computerized Data on Aging, currently sponsored by NIA. The availability of public-use data tapes from national information systems is equally important and, as noted previously, is a subject that requires increased attention.

The panel also recognizes that cross-national and international studies that deal with the elderly can be a valuable source of information. Examination of the characteristics of the elderly in countries with different risks for disease, different lifestyles, and different health care systems contribute to a better understanding of factors that affect health status, utilization, and expenditures for health care of the elderly in the United States. Review of such studies and surveys was beyond the scope of the panel's study; however, this subject is receiving attention. The House Select Committee on Aging conducted a Workshop on Cross-National Data on Aging in October 1985, at which presentations were made by researchers and representatives of government and international organizations conducting studies or surveys of the elderly. The Census Bureau is developing and automating an international data base to permit comparative analyses of demographic social and economic characteristics of many countries, based on their population censuses and surveys. With funds from NIA, the Bureau has been compiling age-specific data on socioeconomic status and mortality among the elderly in a large number of developed and developing countries. The first publication from this project, *An Aging World* (Torrey et al., 1987), provides an overview of trends and a guide to the use of this data base.

Valuable as the three types of data sources discussed are for policy makers, the proving ground for determining the effectiveness of alternative proposals to meet the health care needs of the elderly is demonstration programs with evaluation components. The Health Care Financing Administration has funded projects that test the cost-effectiveness of community-based case management approaches for altering dependence on nursing homes among the elderly and has introduced waivers of restriction in Medicare and Medicaid benefits to assess the value of coordinated long-term care through capitation reimbursement. The Robert Wood Johnson Foundation has provided funds for demonstration programs to address the needs of the health-impaired elderly and, in collaboration with government agencies, the foundation is initiating a project aimed at improving linkages to health and human services, including suitable housing arrangements, for the chronically mentally ill, a significant number of whom are elderly. The Commonwealth Fund has established a Commission on Elderly People Living Alone to assess the health and social problems they face and identify demonstration programs that seek out effective ways to relieve them. Their impact on policy and the diffusion of results are essential features of these efforts, yet national data systems remain the primary sources of information on the changes that occur among the target groups in the population generally.

TABLE 1.1 Panel's Recommendations to Agencies Collecting Data About the Elderly (explanation of acronyms at end of table)

| | Department of Health and Human Services | | | | | | | | | Other Federal Agencies | | | | | |
| | | | | NIH | | | OASH | | | Dept. of Commerce | | | | | |
Chapter Recommendation: Short Title	CDC: NCHS	HCFA	ASPE	NIA	NIMH	All Other NIH	NCHSR OASH	All Other OASH	SSA	Bur. Cen.	Other	Dept. of Labor	IRS	NSF	VA
HEALTH STATUS AND QUALITY OF LIFE															
3.1 Repeat the longitudinal survey of persons of age 55 and over in the NHIS every 5 years.	P														
3.2 Support methodology to increase participation of elderly in health surveys.	x			x			x								
3.3 Include all ages in the NHANES III sample.	x														
3.4 Develop questionnaire for psychiatric disorders of the elderly.	x				x										
3.5 Conduct HANES III follow-up.	x														
3.6 Link health-related surveys to the NDI.	x	x	x	x	x	x		x	x	x					x

P indicates a priority recommendation

39

TABLE 1.1 Continued

Chapter Recommendation: Short Title	CDC: NCHS	HCFA	ASPE	NIA	NIMH	All Other NIH	NCHSR	All Other OASH	SSA	Bur. Cen.	Other	Dept. of Labor	IRS	NSF	VA
3.7 Start surveys of the elderly at age 55.	x	x	x	x	x	x	x	x	x	x					x
3.8 Develop measures of functional status of the elderly.	x			x	x		x								
3.9 Develop measures of productive activity of the elderly.	x		x				x			x		x			
3.10 Include quality-of-life measures in population-based surveys.	x		x	x	x	x	x	x	x	x					x
HEALTH TRANSITION AND THE COMPRESSION OF MORBIDITY															
4.1 Measure physiological characteristics of the elderly over time.	x			x											
4.2 Follow chronically ill populations over time.	x			x		x									

4.3	Develop guidelines for collecting data on co-morbidity.		x	x			
4.4	Include questions in surveys and studies to clarify relationship between disease and disability.	x	x	x	x		
4.5	Study geographic variations in morbidity and mortality risks.	x	x	x	x	x	
4.6	Develop statistical procedures for analysis of multiple data sources on health transitions.	x	x	x	x	x	x
MAINTENANCE OF HEALTH-- PREVENTION OF DISEASE							
5.1	Develop questionnaire items on health promotion and disease prevention for surveys of the elderly.	P	P	P	P	P	
5.2	Add health promotion and disease prevention items to survey of physicians.	x					
5.3*	Study health care personnel requirements for health promotion and disease prevention.	x	x	x			

* Also addressed to Bureau of Health Professions

P indicates a priority recommendation

41

TABLE 1.1 Continued

| | Department of Health and Human Services | | | | | | | | | Other Federal Agencies | | | | | |
| | CDC: | | | NIH | | | OASH | | | Dept. of Commerce | | Dept. of | | | |
Chapter Recommendation: Short Title	NCHS	HCFA	ASPE	NIA	NIMH	All Other NIH	NCHSR	All Other OASH	SSA	Bur. Cen.	Other	Labor	IRS	NSF	VA
QUALITY OF CARE															
6.1 Build on existing data systems to develop quality-of-care measures.	P	P	P	P			P								P
6.2 Link data sets longitudinally to measure quality of care.	x		x				x								
6.3 Conduct research to increase the validity of survey data from elderly respondents.	x			x			x		x	x					
LONG-TERM CARE															
7.1 Develop standard definition of long-term care.								x							

42

7.2	Expand measures of functional disability to include measures of cognitive, social, and emotional functioning.	x			x		
7.3	Continue Longitudinal Study on Aging.	P					
7.4	Increase frequency and expand coverage of the NNHS and supplement with a longitudinal survey.	P					
7.5	Expand coverage of NMFI.	x					
7.6	Develop classification of types of long-term care services.				x		
7.7	Standardize definition of informal supports and collect data on caretakers of the elderly.	x	x	x			
7.8	Use the Long-Term Health Care Minimum Data Set.	x	x	x	x		
7.9	Collect data to measure national expenditures for long-term care.	x	x				x

P indicates a priority recommendation

TABLE 1.1 Continued

Chapter Recommendation: Short Title	Department of Health and Human Services			NIH			OASH			Other Federal Agencies					
	CDC: NCHS	HCFA	ASPE	NIA	NIMH	All Other NIH	NCHSR	All Other OASH	SSA	Dept. of Commerce Bur. Cen.	Other	Dept. of Labor	IRS	NSF	VA
FINANCING OF HEALTH SERVICES FOR THE ELDERLY															
8.1 Publish timely annual estimates of health expenditures for the elderly.		x													
8.2 Augment sample of elderly in future national surveys of medical expenditures.							x								
8.3 Conduct a periodic medical care expenditure survey.	P		P				P								
8.4 Link data for persons ages 55 and older in NMES to administrative records.	P		P				P		P				P		
8.5 Conduct outreach program for NMES data users.			x				x								

44

8.6	Improve release of data from the MSS.	x			
8.7	Improve access to Medicare data for researchers.	P			
8.8	Complete and maintain the MADRS.	P			
8.9	Develop a data system for Medicare utilization under capitated plans.	x			
8.10	Continue studies of the CDHS linked to Medicare files.	x		x	
8.11	Review UHDDS items for disposition of patient.			x	
8.12	Continue the Medicaid Tape-to-Tape Project and provide public use tapes.	x			
8.13	Collect data to estimate economic costs of illness in the elderly by disease.	x	x		x

HEALTH SERVICES UTILIZATION

9.1	Modify national health data systems to reflect changes in service delivery.	P	P	P	P P

P indicates a priority recommendation

45

TABLE 1.1 Continued

	Department of Health and Human Services										Other Federal Agencies					
	CDC:	HCFA	ASPE	NIH			OASH			SSA	Dept. of Commerce		Dept. of Labor	IRS	NSF	VA
Chapter Recommendation: Short Title	NCHS			NIA	NIMH	All Other NIH	NCHSR	OASH	All Other OASH		Bur. Cen.	Other				
9.2 Expand sampling frame for the NAMCS.	x															
9.3 Include dental care utilization items relevant to the elderly in NHANES III.	x															
9.4 Include rehabilitative care questions in surveys.	x	x	x	x				x		x						x
9.5 Explore methods to determine the use of mental health services by the elderly.	x				x			x			x					x
9.6 Link health survey data for elderly to Medicare records.	P	P		P	P	P		P			P					P
9.7 Develop a standard set of items on access to care for surveys of the elderly.	x	x		x	x			x			x					x

46

9.8	Link administrative data for veterans to health surveys.															x
9.9	Oversample rural elderly in health surveys.	x						x								
ENHANCEMENT OF UTILITY OF STATISTICAL SYSTEMS																
10.1	Institutionalize a mechanism for coordinating aging-related statistics.	P	P	P	P	P	P	P	P	P	P	P	P	P	P	P
10.2	Use standard age groups and provide detailed data by age for the elderly.	P	P	P	P	P	P	P	P	P	P		P	P	P	P
10.3	Maintain periodicity of population surveys.	x	x			x		x		x	x		x			
10.4	Include plans for publication and public-use tapes in planning a data system.	P	P	P	P	P		P		P	P		P			P
10.5	Maintain archives of data on aging on a current basis.	x	x	x	x	x		x		x	x					x
10.6	Enhance utility of administrative record systems for statistical purposes.		x							x			x	x		

P indicates a priority recommendation

TABLE 1.1 Continued

Chapter Recommendation: Short Title	Department of Health and Human Services									Other Federal Agencies					
	CDC:			NIH			OASH			Dept. of Commerce		Dept. of			
	NCHS	HCFA	ASPE	NIA	NIMH	All Other NIH	NCHSR	All Other OASH	SSA	Bur. Cen.	Other	Labor	IRS	NSF	VA
10.7 Increase use of data base linkages as source of data on the elderly.	x	x	x	x			x		x	x			x		x
10.8 Augment SIPP sample for the elderly.										x					
10.9 Include health module for the elderly twice in SIPP.										x					
10.10 Develop outreach program for the multiple causes of death file.	x														
10.11 Collect age-sensitive functional disability data in the decennial census.										x					
10.12 Publish more detailed age and geographic data for the elderly from the census.										x					

	1	2	3	4	5	6	7	8	9
10.13 Enhance age detail in the County and City Data Book.				x					
STATISTICAL METHODOLOGY FOR HEALTH POLICY ANALYSIS									
11.1 Conduct methodological research on design and analysis of longitudinal studies.		x		x	x	x	x	x	x
11.2 Explore methods for creation and analysis of linked data bases for the elderly.	x			x	x	x	x	x	x
11.3 Support research on development of improved computerized record linkage systems.	x			x	x	x	x	x	x
11.4 Standardize items useful as matching variables.			x	x	x	x	x	x	x
11.5 Overcome legal and policy obstacles to linkage.	x			x	x	x	x	x	x
11.6 Review data release policy for the CWHS system.			x	x	x		x	x	x
11.7 Develop procedures to permit increased access to microdata files.			x	x	x	x		x	x

P indicates a priority recommendation

TABLE 1.1 Continued

| Chapter Recommendation: Short Title | Department of Health and Human Services | | | | | | | | | Other Federal Agencies | | | | | |
	CDC: NCHS	HCFA	ASPE	NIH NIA	NIMH	All Other NIH	OASH NCHSR	All Other OASH	SSA	Dept. of Commerce Bur. Cen.	Other	Dept. of Labor	IRS	NSF	VA
11.8 Establish an expanded program of decennial population projections.										x					
11.9 Project mortality rates by cause, age, race, and sex for use in population projections.									x						
11.10 Release tapes of population projections.				x					x	x					
11.11 Document the nature of uncertainty for population projections.				x					x	x				x	
11.12 Study methodological and data requirements for forecasts of the aging population.				P					P	P				P	
11.13 Support research on methods for conducting and reporting policy analysis.	x	x	x						x	x		x	x		x

50

*"All other OASH" includes Office of Disease Prevention/Health Promotion and the National Committee on Vital and Health Statistics, which is advisory to the secretary of HHS but reports through the assistant secretary for health.

ACRONYMS

ASPE	Assistant Secretary for Planning and Evaluation
Bur. Cen.	Bureau of the Census
CDC	Centers for Disease Control
CDHS	Continuous Disability History Sample
CMHS	Continuous Medicare History Sample
HCFA	Health Care Financing Administration
IRS	Internal Revenue Service
MADRS	Medicare Automated Data Retrieval System
MSS	Medicare Statistical System
NAMCS	National Ambulatory Medical Care Survey
NCHS	National Center for Health Statistics
NCHSR	National Center for Health Services Research and Health Care Technology Assessment

NDI	National Death Index
NHANES III	National Health and Nutrition Examination Survey
NIA	National Institute of Aging
NIH	National Institutes of Health
NIMH	National Institute of Mental Health
NMES	National Medical Expenditure Survey
NMFI	National Master Facility Inventory
NNHS	National Nursing Home Survey
NSF	National Science Foundation
OASH	Office of Assistant Secretary for Health
SSA	Social Security Administration
UHDDS	Uniform Hospital Discharge Data Set
VA	Veterans Administration

2
Social, Economic, and Demographic Changes Among the Elderly

The population of the United States is growing older, a phenomenon widely noted and described, with significant implications for the nation's health, social, and economic institutions. It is necessary to understand the past demographic and socioeconomic trends to better estimate the future size and characteristics of the older population as well as to forecast their demand for services and the extent to which those demands can be met. Analysis of the demographic and socioeconomic trends of the elderly population will also help identify data needed to make informed policy decisions related to the health of the future elderly population.

THE CHANGING DEMOGRAPHIC STRUCTURE OF THE POPULATION

The distribution of the population in the United States has shifted rapidly in both the number and proportion of the population age 65 and over. This subgroup has grown faster than the rest of the population in recent decades, will continue to grow at a more rapid rate for the remainder of the twentieth century, and is expected to continue to increase well into the next century. Between 1950 and 1980 the population age 65 and older more than doubled, from 12.3 million in 1950 to 25.5 million in 1980 (Taeuber, 1983). During this 30-year period, the percentage increase in the number of elderly was 74 percent larger than for the population under age 65—108 percent compared with 62 percent. For the oldest-old, age 85 and over, the rise was the largest, a 281 percent increase from 577,000 in 1950 to 2.2 million in 1980.

Population Forecasts

The size of the elderly population today and in the near future is relatively simple to estimate: it depends on the births in the early years of this century and the deaths in the birth cohort in subsequent years. (A small portion of the total elderly population is accounted for by net migration, which is not as accurately counted as births and deaths.) The elderly population in the next century depends on the births beginning in the 1930s and the estimated deaths in each year's birth cohort. These estimates are subject to increasing uncertainty as we move further into the future.

Birth rates were relatively high in the early part of this century, low in 1920-1940, high in the postwar years 1946-1964, lower again in 1965-1973, and slightly higher in more recent years. Throughout, there have been important variations by age of mother, birth order, and race. Death rates, meanwhile, have declined or remained level throughout the twentieth century, although at rates that varied by age, race, and sex. Declines in mortality rates have been consistently greater for women than for men and, since 1968, almost as large for the oldest-old as for young-old (ages 65-74) females. Current indications are that the declines in mortality rates are continuing (National Center for Health Statistics, 1986a). The future population has been estimated by the Bureau of the Census on the basis of a completed cohort fertility of 1.9 births per woman and a continued decline in mortality rates. The most likely forecasts are identified as the Bureau's "middle series," which are the basis for the analysis in this report. Should there be great advances in medical care or unpredictable epidemics, the estimated size of the elderly population might be considerably different.

Table 2.1 shows the actual and projected growth of the older population. The middle series estimates a steady rise in the elderly (age 65 and over), from 25.5 million in 1980 (11.3 percent of the total population) to a projected 64.3 million (21.1 percent) in 2030—more than doubling over the 50-year period. The number of oldest-old will continue to grow rapidly in the next 50 years, from 2.2 million in 1980, to 8.8 million in 2030, and to 16.1 million in 2050. The progression of the postwar baby-boom cohort, those born from 1946 to 1964 (Siegel and Davidson, 1984) may be seen in the peak for

TABLE 2.1 Actual and Projected Growth of the Older Population, 1980-2050 (numbers in millions)

Year	Total Population	65-74 years		75-84 years		85 years and over		65 years and over	
		No.	%	No.	%	No.	%	No.	%
1980	226.5	15.6	6.9	7.7	3.4	2.2	1.0	25.5	11.3
1990	250.0	18.0	7.2	10.3	4.1	3.5	1.4	31.8	12.7
2000	268.0	17.7	6.6	12.2	4.6	5.1	1.9	35.0	13.1
2010	283.1	20.3	7.2	12.2	4.3	6.8	2.4	39.3	13.9
2020	296.3	29.8	10.2	14.3	4.8	7.3	2.5	51.4	17.3
2030	304.3	34.4	11.3	21.1	6.9	8.8	2.9	64.3	21.1
2040	308.0	29.2	9.5	24.5	8.0	12.9	4.2	66.6	21.6
2050	308.9	30.0	9.7	21.0	6.8	16.1	5.2	67.1	21.7

Source: Taeuber (1983).

the 65-74 age group in 2030, for the 75-84 age group in 2040, and those age 85 and over in 2050. The oldest-old population group was 1 percent of the total population and 9 percent of the elderly in 1980; by 2050, this group is projected to increase to 5 percent of the total population and 24 percent of the elderly.

The accelerated growth within the elderly population of those age 85 and over has shifted attention to this subgroup and its unique set of needs. The oldest-old are at risk for chronic illness, tend to be functionally dependent, and have greater needs for medical, social, and support services.

Forecasts by Sex

At birth, every cohort has a small excess of males but, owing to the higher death rates for the male population and the more rapid improvement in mortality for women, there is a large excess of women at older ages. In 1980 there were 10.2 million elderly men (age 65 and over) and 15.2 elderly women, a ratio of 68 men to 100 women. The Census Bureau population projections show that the sex ratio of the population age 65 and over will continue to fall in the next few decades, but more slowly than in the past, reaching 64 males per 100 females in the year 2000 (Siegel and Davidson, 1984). Subsequently, the trend will change, so that by the year 2020 the sex ratio of the elderly population will be 69 men per 100 females.

The sex ratio declines rapidly with increasing age: in 1980 there were 80 males per 100 females for those age 65-69 and 44 males per 100 females for those age 85 and older. For the latter group, the ratio of men to women is projected to fall between 1980 and 2020, from 44 men to 36 per 100 women. Since the vast majority of the oldest-old are female, many of the health, social, and economic problems of this group are those of women.

Forecasts by Race

In 1980, 12 percent of the white population was age 65 and older—a much larger proportion than the 8 percent of the black population (Siegel and Davidson, 1984). The Census Bureau attributes the difference to higher fertility of the black population and secondarily to higher mortality at ages below 65. The Census Bureau projects that the black population of the future will continue to be a younger population than the white, although improvements in mortality rates for elderly blacks are expected. By 2020, 19 percent of the total white population compared with 12 percent of the black population is projected to be age 65 and over (U.S. Department of Health and Human Services, 1985b).

Geographic Distribution of the Elderly Population

Older persons tend to move far less often than younger persons, remaining in the state, county, or local area where they settled during their adult years. Between 1975 and 1979, their rate of interstate migration was 3.6 percent (Bureau of the Census, 1984). Between 1970 and 1980, the largest numerical increases in elderly people were in the states of Florida, California, and Texas. Growth of more than 50 percent in the number of elderly in that decade occurred in Arizona, Florida, Nevada, New Mexico, Alaska, and Hawaii. In 1980, almost half the elderly were living in eight states: California, Florida, New York, Pennsylvania, Texas, Illinois, Ohio, and Michigan, but these states also accounted for 47.9 percent of the total population. In Florida, 17.3 percent of its 1980 population was elderly, the highest proportion of any state, although Florida had only 4.3 percent of the total population (Taeuber, 1983).

Short-term population projections to the year 2000 by the Bureau of the Census show significant differences in rates of change in the population of the four regions of the United States. The West and South will be the fastest-growing regions from 1980 to 2000, increasing 45 percent and 31 percent, respectively. The North Central region is projected to lose population during the same period. The elderly population in all regions, however, is projected to rise, ranging from a 12 percent increase in the Northeast to a 60 percent increase in the South and West (Taeuber, 1983).

These geographic data imply differential use of medical care services by region. For example, in the Northeast and North Central regions, the number of nursing home beds will need to increase by 44 percent. In the South and West, the number of nursing home beds will have to more than double to meet the needs of the projected elderly population (Rice, 1985).

Marital Status and Living Arrangements

Among the most important social characteristics affecting the welfare of the elderly are those that pertain to their marital status and living arrangements. Elderly men are most likely to be married; elderly women are most likely to be widowed. In 1981, 79 percent of elderly men and 39 percent of elderly women were married. For elderly women, the proportion of widows increases rapidly and remains at a high level: for the 65-74 age group, 40 percent are widowed; for the group age 75 and older, 68 percent are widowed.

Marital status has a direct bearing on the living arrangements of the elderly. Among elderly men, 82 percent live in a family setting and more than 74 percent are married and living with their wives. A very different situation exists for elderly women; 55 percent live in a family setting and only 36 percent are married and living with their husbands. In short, women age 65 and older are more likely to be widowed than married and living alone rather than with husbands. The number of elderly women living alone has doubled in the last 15 years, and projections by the Census Bureau show a substantial increase up to 1995 in the proportion of households with an elderly female living alone or with nonrelatives (Siegel and Davidson, 1984).

This trend has important implications for housing needs and the demand for institutional care. With the decline in the proportion of the elderly living with relatives likely to continue, there will probably be a greater need for the provision of social support and health services by the community or other public sources.

Education

The level of educational attainment of the elderly population is currently less than that of the younger population. This educational gap by age group has narrowed since 1950 and is expected to nearly close in the next decade, due to increased compulsory secondary school requirements, as well as educational opportunities made available by the G.I. bill after World War II. A lower proportion of foreign-born in the future elderly population due to changes in immigration will also serve to increase the educational attainment of the elderly population. The greater education of the future elderly population implies a change in demand for services: combined with rising income, they may seek and demand more and better health care and other programs for their needs (Rosenwaike, 1985).

Income

The income of the elderly has improved over time. According to the Congressional Budget Office, "After accounting for inflation, the average cash income of families with elderly members increased by nearly 18 percent during the 15-year period from 1969 to 1984, the latest year for which detailed data are available—while the average income of unrelated elderly individuals rose by 34 percent" (Gordon, 1986:2). The income of younger families also rose in this period, but not as much as for the elderly. Average elderly family income was 68 percent of average nonelderly family income in 1969 and 78 percent in 1984. For unrelated individuals, the elderly-to-nonelderly income ratio was 50 percent in 1969 and 60 percent in 1984.

The poverty rate among the elderly also declined in 1969-1984, from 25 percent to 12 percent, but in 1984 an additional 9 percent of the elderly had incomes of not more than 25 percent above the poverty level. In 1984 incomes were below the poverty level for 9 percent of elderly men, 15 percent of elderly women, and 36 percent of elderly black women.

Social Security benefits are the largest single source of money income for the elderly (nearly 40 percent), followed by earnings, ...me. and private and public pensions. The most sig- .... for the elderly population since . importance of earnings and an .come from Social Security, public .. Noncash benefits are estimated , of the elderly, the most important .d, food stamps, and publicly owned .ugh asset ownership (including savings and home ownership) is fairly common at the time of retirement, the value of assets owned by the elderly is low.

Current expenditures by the elderly are highest for shelter, followed by food, transportation, and health care, which, surprisingly, uses less of the budget than transportation. These expenditures must be considered along with available economic resources in planning and developing public policies for the elderly.

Labor Force Participation

Sharp declines have occurred in the last few decades in the labor force participation of men age 65 and older: from a third in 1960, to a quarter in 1970, to 17.6 percent in 1981 (U.S. Congress, Senate, 1986a). This trend is associated with an increase in voluntary early retirement and a drop in self-employment. With the growth in retirement programs, more older workers have been financially able to retire earlier. Projections by the Bureau of Labor Statistics (BLS) show a continued decline in labor force participation of elderly men at least up to 2000 (Fullerton, 1980). The proportion of older women in the labor force has increased moderately since 1960, due to economic necessity, more education, changes in social roles, and increased divorce rates that result in more women heading their own households. BLS projections show a moderate decline in the labor force participation of women age 65 and older and a continued increase for women age 55-64 up to 2000 (Siegel and Davidson, 1984).

Part-time employment is now an increasingly important source of employment for the elderly: half of those age 65 and over who work do so on a part-time basis, up from a third in 1960. Age at retirement and labor force participation of the elderly have a direct effect on retirement programs and economic dependency. The age of eligibility for Social Security and other pension benefits will affect the age of retirement for many elderly, which in turn affects their level of income and economic dependency. The projected decline in labor force participation rates of older persons will lead to a continued rise in the ratio of older nonworkers to the working population and an associated increased dependency. The Social Security Act of 1983 advanced the age of retirement from 65 to 67 for payment of full benefits. The change is to be phased in from age 65 in 1983, to 66 in 2006, to 67 in 2027. It is uncertain what effect the law will have on actual age at retirement.

Dependency Ratio

The social support systems now in place reflect the current balance between the size of the working population and the retired. The trends for people to live longer and for families to have fewer children are changing the shape of the elderly dependency ratio—the population age 65 and over divided by the population ages 18-64, the working population. This ratio has risen steadily, from 11 per 100 in 1940 to 19 per 100 in 1980, and it is expected to reach 22 in 2010. The expected leveling off or slower increase in the next several decades will be followed by a sharp increase between 2010 and 2030, when the baby-boom cohorts will reach old age; the ratio is expected to be 29 per 100 by 2020 and 37 per 100 by 2030 (Siegel and Davidson, 1984). At the same time, projected low fertility rates will result in fewer young persons and, thus, a declining young dependency ratio, defined as the population under age 18 divided by the working population, ages 18-64.

The total dependency ratio, the sum of the young and elderly ratios, is a crude index of the total burden on the working population of its support of both old and young dependents. The total dependency ratio has declined since 1960, but it is expected to increase in the next century, and the increase in the elderly dependency ratio will be greater than the decline in the young dependency ratio. The elderly are primarily supported by publicly funded programs while, except for public education, mostly private (i.e., family) funds support the young. Since the elderly will be the most rapidly growing age group and more costly, the change in the dependency ratios will be a major policy issue for both Social Security and the hospital insurance programs under Medicare that are financed by payroll taxes (Rice and Feldman, 1983).

In addition to the unknown effects of advancing the age of retirement to 67 for payment of full benefits, fully effective in 2027, other social and legislative changes in the next 50 years may change the relationships between the working and the retired populations, significantly changing the elderly dependency ratio.

Morbidity Patterns

There is considerable conjecture and controversy regarding future morbidity patterns. One theory holds that the improvements in lifestyle will delay the onset of disability and will result in a reduction in the prevalence of morbidity from chronic disease and a compression of morbidity at older ages. This theory foresees a continuing decline in premature death and the emergence of a pattern of natural death at the end of a natural life span (Fries, 1980). Another theory argues that chronic disease prevalence and disability will increase as life expectancy increases, leading to a pandemic of mental disorders and chronic diseases (Kramer, 1980). This theory projects that the extension of life is bringing an extension of disease and disability. The increases in the prevalence of chronic conditions due to medical technology have been called the failures of success (Gruenberg, 1977).

A recent review of the evidence (Schneider and Brody, 1983) concludes that the number of very old people is increasing rapidly, the average period of diminished vigor will probably rise, chronic disease will probably occupy a larger proportion of people's life spans, and the needs for medical care in later life are likely to increase substantially. Models linking morbidity and mortality can be developed to predict how healthy or ill cohorts of the older population will be in the future (Manton, 1982).

THE LIMITATIONS OF AVAILABLE DATA

Needs for data in several areas related to the demographic and socioeconomic trends described can be identified. The sources of currently available demographic and socioeconomic data on the aging population are the decennial census and sample surveys, including the Current Population Survey (CPS), the Survey of Income and Program Participation (SIPP), and the National Health Interview Survey (NHIS). These surveys have sample sizes that are too small to provide detailed age breaks and characteristics of subgroups of the elderly population. Analytic studies of the oldest-old, for example, are severely hampered because the size of the sample age 85 and older in these surveys is not large enough to provide a socioeconomic profile of this growing segment of the elderly. Future planning to meet the needs of this age group, especially the need for institutional care, will require more in-depth knowledge of the sex, race, marital composition, and living arrangements of the oldest-old, along with a more detailed income and wealth profile than is currently available from survey statistics. A major requirement is to obtain a large-enough sample of the elderly to provide detailed age and subgroup characteristics.

Detailed data on income, wealth, and pension statistics for the elderly are essential for policy analysis. Better income measures—for example, the use of income distributions rather than averages—are needed to more accurately assess the economic status of the older population. Noncash benefits also need to be quantified in determining the financial well-being of elderly persons. And since employment status has a direct bearing on economic resources, various measures of income should separate the older population into working versus retired categories. In addition to income and wealth data, there is a need for data on detailed pension programs and retirement income. A related issue is the need to analyze retirement trends in terms of a measure such as the average age at retirement. Better income data and measures will provide a more accurate picture of the financial well-being and economic resources of the elderly and also aid in planning public and private retirement, health, and social programs. Methods of forecasting income at the time of retirement also need to be developed with those planning efforts.

Limited data are now available on the pension prospects of women. Due to women's increased labor force participation, the situation of women as they turn 65 in future years is likely to be quite different in terms of anticipated future income and pension coverage and benefits. In order to forecast the pensions of women, there is a need to monitor the pension benefits being accrued by the more recent cohorts of women.

The increased labor force participation of women implies greater financial prospects from pension benefits on one hand, and lesser availability to provide a caregiver role for age parents on the other. With the rapid growth of the oldest-old, there is a greater likelihood for the young-old to have extremely aged parents in need of care. Fewer women will be available to provide such support and greater reliance will shift to formal caregiver and support systems.

Forecasts of the older population are especially useful for long-range planning, and several types of demographic and socioeconomic data are needed for more accurate and useful projections of the elderly. First, greater age detail at extreme ages (i.e., over 75 or 80 years) is needed, which would allow analysis of such factors as institutionalization (Myers, 1985). Second, forecasts of the living arrangements and future housing needs of the elderly are needed to aid in planning efforts in the areas of publicly subsidized housing and institutional facilities. Projections of both the noninstitutionalized and institutionalized long-term care populations are needed.

Data on ethnicity and the foreign-born population of the elderly have been largely ignored. Although the proportion of foreign-born elderly persons is expected to decline in future years, the need to study changes in the foreign-born composition of the older population arises due in part to different needs of such subgroups.

Greater geographic detail in national projections is also needed, along with forecasts of migratory flows of the elderly (Myers, 1985). Better data are needed on migration and mobility of the elderly and the subsequent population redistribution, which is especially valuable in projection work. The need to better forecast migratory flows for states and local areas coincides with the need to know about the concentration or distribution of the elderly population. The following questions become increasingly important for regional planning and the provision of health and social services: Will there be a residential turnover among the elderly, from central cities to suburban areas? What is the likelihood of certain suburbs' becoming essentially elderly communities? Information related to such questions can help regional planners decide where to put facilities such as nursing homes and board and care homes. Knowledge about interstate migration as well as residential mobility of the elderly is important for projection purposes.

Short-term projections (to 2000) show a regional shift among the elderly from the Northeast and North Central regions to the South and West regions. In a detailed study of migration patterns of the elderly based on decennial census data, Longino observed that even while migration into the sunbelt states continued, outmigrants from Florida to northern states were characterized by high proportions of persons age 75 and over returning to their state of birth (Longino et al., 1984). Study of migration streams by age can contribute to more accurate projections, and thereby to better state and regional planning.

The population ages 45-64 today will become the "new aged" population in the next 20 years, and longitudinal data are needed to monitor this group. These cohorts require special attention, as they represent cohorts very different from the current elderly population in terms of educational, marital, income, and perhaps health characteristics (Myers, 1985). Changes in composition, behavior, and needs of the future elderly can best be foreseen by analyzing the differences between newly entering cohorts of the elderly and their immediate predecessors (Serow and Sly, 1985). Serow contends that the group ages 55-64 in 1980 is critically different in composition and life-course experiences, separating the elderly of yesterday from the elderly of the future. This leads to several implications for the later years of life for the new aged. The future elderly are also expected to have relatively higher incomes and greater assets, along with better health. On the basis of the changes in the labor force experiences of women noted earlier, future generations of women can be expected to enter their retirement years with greater financial resources, from their own pension and Social Security entitlements, but with fewer familial resources to provide necessary support. Although tomorrow's elderly may have an improved financial position, the size of the future population will increase the need for long-term home care and may require a greater supporting role by society. As the elderly population ages, the number of nursing home residents is projected to increase by 60 percent by 2003.

Successive cohorts of the elderly are projected to have both increased educational attainment and higher incomes. As educational level has been shown to be associated with various measures of health status as well as demands for better health care, it becomes increasingly important to study the implications of a more highly educated older population. Higher income levels of tomorrow's elderly imply a greater ability to pay for better health care for acute conditions. Data on changing conditions for future generations of the elderly also need to incorporate the implications of housing and transportation available to the elderly, as these factors affect people's quality of life, which in turn affects measures of health and illness.

Related to data needs on the older population are several methodological issues. These areas include the development of appropriate health status measures for major socioeconomic surveys, the linkage of data bases, the need for longitudinal studies of socioeconomic and health characteristics of the elderly, and studies of the elderly on an age cohort basis.

Appropriate health measures need to be developed and incorporated into the major socioeconomic surveys. We need new approaches to the development of measures of physical, cognitive, emotional, and social functioning. Several measures are available and have been used in national surveys. These need to be improved and broadened to take into account the positive or successful aspects as well as the negative aspects of aging and to reflect ordinary behaviors and activities of older persons that indicate their quality of life and affect their relationships with those close to them (National Research Council, 1986).

Longitudinal studies of socioeconomic and health characteristics of the elderly are especially relevant. Such data are essential for assessment of transitions over the life cycle. Despite the physiologic losses and psychosocial stresses often associated with advanced age, many elderly individuals have the vitality and resilience to function effectively or to recover and function independently, once again, following a disabling condition. Data are needed that measure the extent to which older individuals remain in good health and the changes that occur as they move from one state of health to another, whether this marks an improvement or progressive loss of function leading to disability, dependency and, ultimately, mortality. Measuring this requires repeated observations on the same people over time, i.e., longitudinal information on both the well and the impaired in the population (National Research Council, 1986).

Data for the elderly on an age cohort basis are needed in addition to those being collected on an age period basis. For example, the onset of a particular disease or condition could vary by birth cohort. Analysis of data on a cohort basis would thus reveal if a shift in the age of onset has occurred for successive cohorts. Such data would aid greatly in understanding tomorrow's elderly.

Data base linkage could be invaluable to research on the elderly. Separate analyses have been conducted based on survey data, medical records, and administrative data. By linking these sources, more detailed analyses will be possible along with the testing of new relationships. For example, linking Medicare files with social survey data and medical records could provide information on Medicare use by the availability of a social network or by the severity of the medical condition. Such linkage could supply a more comprehensive health profile of the elderly.

IMPLICATIONS FOR THE STUDY

The social, economic, and demographic changes in successive cohorts of elderly people highlighted in this chapter have implications for the topics discussed in each of the chapters in this report. Indeed, they helped determine the topics selected for discussion.

3
Health Status and Quality of Life

As individuals age, they are at risk for diseases and disabling conditions, use more medical care services, and incur medical expenses. While there is no doubt that age is a predictor of morbidity and mortality, its predictive value is limited. The health status of the elderly is better than generally assumed, varies remarkably among individuals, and is changing as successive cohorts progressively challenge the definition of old age.

One major misconception in the health care field is that the elderly are a homogeneous group of frail individuals progressing rapidly toward needs for long-term care. The elderly actually are a very heterogeneous group. It has been noted that as individuals age, they become less like each other (Rowe, 1985). From a physiological perspective, differences between individuals characteristically increase with advancing age in those factors that change with age, such as blood glucose level and blood pressure. From a clinical perspective, specific subgroups of elderly individuals can be identified, including the 5 percent who at any one time are residing in long-term care facilities and the larger portion who have major functional declines. The marked effect of age itself on disability, morbidity, and mortality has led many workers in the field to divide the overall elderly population into at least two groups, a young-old population and an old-old population, which is characterized by frailty and marked increases in the need for acute and long-term care services (Besdine, 1982). These clear age-related differences suggest the value of collecting different types of data in different age subsets. The panel has chosen to use three age subsets: young-old (age 65-74), old (age 75-84), and oldest-old (age 85 and older).

The health care of elderly persons, perhaps more than any other age group, is influenced by the social support system available to them (Brody, 1981). The network of current and potential informal supports, such as family or friends, has an important role in modulating the clinical impact of underlying disease and is often the major determinant in decisions to institutionalize elderly people. For every impaired elderly person in a nursing home, there are approximately two equally impaired elderly people living in the community who often can remain there by virtue of the critical role of informal support systems, which provide approximately 80 percent of their long-term care (Doty, 1986).

In choosing which data need to be collected and how they should be analyzed, it is important to recognize that the needs of the elderly differ from those of younger individuals, not only from a quantitative perspective (i.e., the elderly use more health care services), but also qualitatively. "Just as children are not merely young versions of adults, the elderly are not simply old adults. They require special approaches" (Rowe, 1985:827) and their health care needs reflect a complex interaction of the physiologic changes with age, their psychosocial concomitants, and the various pathologic processes that occur with advancing frequency in senescence.

Although health status per se is not a policy issue, policy analysts need to be able to detect trends and to forecast changes among the elderly in their health status and utilization of services. Development of such trend data requires a stable program of periodic surveys of the health status of the elderly population.

This chapter reviews and summarizes what is known about the elderly and the aging process in the later years with respect to health status, functional status, and quality of life and their determinants. The major sources of statistics relevant to these topics are reviewed and changes are recommended that will augment the available information on the health status of the elderly, provide information to understand the health needs of the elderly, provide a dynamic description of aging as a process, and lead to improved measures of functional status of the active elderly that will help trace the transitions from their well state to states of disability as well as measure their need for assistance. The chapter concludes with a review of the relationship between health and functional status and the quality of life experienced by the elderly and discusses some of the components of quality of life with emphasis on the relationship between productive activity and quality of life.

HEALTH STATUS

Characteristics of Health Status and Data

Successful Aging

For too long, gerontological research has focused on the losses in function that occur with advancing age. We have lost sight of the fact that most elderly individuals function very well and report their health as good or excellent. Despite the physiologic losses and the psychosocial stresses often associated with advanced age, many elderly individuals have the vitality and resilience to function at a high level. Data collection should take into account the positive aspects of aging rather than purely functional decline, disease, and mortality. Similarly, there needs to be increasing recognition of the capacity of individuals to improve over time; thus, data sets should be conceptualized with a view to following individuals as they increase in their functioning, rather than only to their entering a pathway of progressive loss of function leading to disability and ultimate mortality.

Longevity Extension and Compression of Morbidity

A major policy issue relates to the relationship between changes in the mortality experience of the elderly population and coincident changes in the underlying morbidity and disability experiences.

In 1900, a man who reached the age of 65 could expect to live 11 more years, and a woman age 65 could expect to live 12 more years. By 1984, men turning 65 could expect to live 14.5 more years, and women turning 65 could expect to live 18.7 more years (National Center for Health Statistics, 1986c). This "longevity revolution" has even affected the very old, as the past two decades have brought dramatic reductions in mortality rates among those over 80, both men and women.

The important issue, however, is the quality of the additional years of life for the elderly. Are the additional years ones of vigor and independence, or of frailty and dependence? Will future increases in longevity be associated with prolongation of dependency or will active life expectancy increase ("compression of morbidity") as health promotion and disease prevention strategies become increasingly effective (Rowe, 1985)?

"The initial claim that as mortality declines morbidity will also decline has recently been challenged by studies suggesting that the increased life span of the old-old is not accompanied by decreased morbidity and may actually result in more dramatic increases in the need for health care services" (Rowe, 1985:828). While federal statistics have documented the changes in life epollutantsxpectancy during the twentieth century, there are no national data showing whether the period of vitality has also changed. Thus, it is not known whether either the actual number or the proportion of people's later years that are spent in a healthy state has increased, remained the same, or decreased during the period when the life span has increased. Chapter 4 discusses this issue in detail.

Transitions from Morbidity to Disability and Mortality

The World Health Organization has proposed a model (Manton, 1986a) that describes the linkages between mortality, disability, and morbidity (discussed in detail in Chapter 4). While it is clear that the overall mortality experience of the elderly population has an underlying curve of morbidity experience in which individuals accumulate diseases and losses in specific capabilities, the specific interactions between the development of diseases and the subsequent development of disability have not been elucidated. It is particularly important to recognize that many different pathologic processes may result in, or contribute to, identical functional impairments. For any particular person, several coincident pathologic processes interact in a complex fashion to result in disability. This interaction is often strongly influenced by other factors, particularly in the psychosocial sphere.

The marked variability in health status among the elderly and the uncertain nature of the link between the presence of pathological processes, their functional consequences, and eventual mortality underlie the importance of an approach to the elderly that permits analysis of the transitions that individuals make from one functional status or health state to another. It is clearly inadequate to focus only on mortality, hospitalization, or institutionalization as end points and increasingly important to detect changes in function when they occur and to develop sensitive measures of the severity of disease processes. It is particularly important in studies of transitions in health status to maintain a perspective that permits detection of improvements over time, rather than just losses in functions.

This approach may be more difficult in elderly patients than in their younger counterparts because there appears to be a very short recall period for health interactions in the elderly. In addition, self-reported data regarding some functional status measures, such as those referred to as instrumental activities of daily living, may not be adequate. Studies should be carried out to clarify whether the inaccuracy of such self-report data is a function of age or age-associated diseases, such as those that impair cognitive function.

The Need for Acute and Chronic Care

Over the past several years, the dramatic increase in Medicaid spending for nursing home care has led to a progressive interest in the long-term care needs of the elderly and to finding alternatives to high-cost institutionalization. The critical importance of acute care in the elderly appears to have been underemphasized: more than 40 percent of the health care expenditures of the elderly are for acute care (Waldo and Lazenby, 1984). In addition, the common practice of identifying the type of care given by the site in which it is given is increasingly misleading. On one hand, many elderly individuals in acute care facilities receive chronic care. Some are admitted to an acute care hospital in order to gain access to a long-term care facility, and some are admitted to a hospital because of a worsening of a chronic condition. On the other hand, with the implementation of prospective payment and diagnosis-related groups under Medicare, there is a tendency for acute care hospitals to discharge patients to long-term care facilities earlier than they did previously. Many nursing homes are now faced with providing acute care, especially acute postoperative care, in facilities not designed for this care and by staffs who are often inadequately trained. In tracking patients' progress through the health care system, it is becoming increasingly important to know not only the locus in which care is provided, but also the specific nature of the care.

Determinants of Disease in Old Age

With advancing age, the general tendency is a shift from acute to chronic diseases. For example, hypertension and coronary heart disease increase with age, as does the risk of cancer, autoimmune diseases such as pernicious anemia and Addison's disease, and diseases of the bones and joints such as arthritis and osteoporosis.

The reasons for such increases are not fully understood. Increases in specific disease categories may reflect increased vulnerability with age, in turn caused by a wide range of age-related phenomena, from reduction of the immune functions to losses in physical agility. But age-related increases in pathology do not necessarily imply increased inherent vulnerability; they can also result from cumulative exposure to environmental pollutants or from reduced resources, both economic and interpersonal. Per capita income decreases with age, especially after work and retirement, and the likelihood of personal loss through bereavement increases, with possible concomitant reduction in sources of health-promotive assistance and support.

To the risk-enhancing aspects of old age must be added characteristics or capabilities of the elderly that may decrease risk. Each successive age group consists by definition of survivors, so there is an inevitable selection factor at work. Separate from the constitutional or genetic factors in such selection are the effects of learning. With increasing age people may be differentially successful in learning to recognize their own limits, avoid various environmental risk factors (e.g., quit smoking), or modify the severity of the risk (e.g., smoke less). Such learning then becomes a counterforce to the age-related factors that increase risk of disease and death.

Current understanding of these complexities is fragmentary. For example, some demographic characteristics are known to be associated with longevity (i.e., negatively related to standardized mortality ratios), but the causal pathways or the reasons that these relationships become weaker with age is not known. Such reductions in the older age groups have been observed for education, socioeconomic level of residence, race, and marital status. Some predictive relationships (e.g., the effect of high blood pressure on mortality and morbidity and the effect of supportive social ties on the risk of hospitalization), however, persist throughout the entire age range. And some relationships (e.g., the effect of marital dissatisfaction on coronary heart disease) seem to increase with age.

Special Characteristics of Illness Behavior in the Elderly*

Underreporting of Health Conditions

An important characteristic underlying functional impairment in the elderly is the failure of many persons to seek assistance despite the fact that both clear-cut illnesses and abnormalities are present. Studies in several countries with varying health care systems indicate that symptoms of serious and treatable diseases often go unreported (Rowe, 1983; Anderson, 1966). Health problems reported by frail elderly persons are thus frequently only the tip of the iceberg of treatable conditions. As Besdine (1982) pointed out, nonreporting of symptoms of underlying disease in elderly persons is an especially dangerous phenomenon when coupled with the passive structure of American health care delivery, which lacks prevention-oriented or early detection efforts. He notes that aged persons, burdened by society's and their own views of functional loss with aging, cannot be relied on to initiate appropriate health care for themselves, especially early in the course of an illness.

Multiple Pathology

The coexistence of several diseases has a profoundly negative influence on health and functional independence in the elderly, and the number of pathologic conditions in a person is strongly related to age. Elderly persons who live in the community have on the average three to four important disabilities (Anderson, 1966), and the hospitalized elderly have evidence of six pathologic conditions (Wilson et al., 1962). The entire array of diseases present in an individual patient must be considered as models are developed to describe pathways to dependency and as treatment plans are developed. Multiple pathology has obvious implications for health interview surveys, provider surveys, hospital discharge records, and the vital statistics on cause of death.

Atypical or Altered Presentation of Disease

A fundamental principle of geriatric medicine is that many diseases have signs and symptoms in the elderly that differ from those

---

*This section closely parallels the section on "Illness Behavior in the Elderly" in Rowe (1985:830).

in their younger counterparts. These alterations can take two major forms. First, specific symptoms characteristic of a disease in middle age may be replaced by other symptoms in old age. For instance, in acute myocardial infarction, some studies have suggested that elderly persons are less likely than younger adults to have chest pain. But acute myocardial infarction is not "silent" in older persons, who have instead a variety of other acute signs and symptoms. The second difference is that elderly persons may have nonspecific signs and symptoms, such as confusion, weakness, weight loss, or "failure to thrive" instead of specific symptoms indicating the organ or system affected.

HEALTH DATA

Major Sources of Health Statistics

The United States is fortunate in having well-developed systems of data collection for demographic, social, and economic characteristics of the population and for its rates of morbidity and mortality, health expenditures, and utilization. These data collections are the major responsibility of two agencies: the Bureau of the Census in the Department of Commerce and the National Center for Health Statistics (NCHS) in the Department of Health and Human Services. Many other agencies collect data directly related to their missions.

The two major agencies produce general-purpose data for program and policy decisions and devote a substantial portion of their staff to serve needs of researchers and policy makers and the general public. Historically, the programs of the National Center for Health Statistics have been the major source of information on the health status of the population. This report, in its discussion of policy issues related to health problems of the elderly, draws on only a small part of the data available on the health of the U.S. population. The surveys relevant to this chapter are the National Health and Nutrition Examination Survey and the National Health Interview Survey and its supplements. A related source of information is the series of national medical expenditure surveys conducted by the National Center for Health Services Research and Health Care Technology Assessment in 1977, 1980, and 1987, which are discussed in detail in Chapters 8 and 9 (on financing and utilization of health services). Recently a new source of health status information became available from the Bureau of the Census: in 1984 the Bureau fielded the first wave of the Survey on Income and Program Participation (SIPP), which includes a topical module on health and disability. Although health status is not its major focus, SIPP does provide data that can be used to relate health status to income; SIPP is discussed in detail in Chapter 10.

The National Health Interview Survey

The National Health Interview Survey is a principal source of information on the health of the civilian, noninstitutionalized population of the United States. The survey, conducted continuously since 1957, provides national data annually on the incidence of acute illness and accidental injuries, the prevalence of chronic conditions and impairments, the extent of disability, the utilization of health care services, and other health-related topics.

The data are obtained from 40,000 household interviews that include about 110,000 persons. Of these, 7,500 to 8,500 are ages 65-74, and 4,800 to 5,400 are age 75 and older. Because of budget constraints the sample size was reduced by 50 percent in 1986. To provide data on special topic areas in addition to the basic NHIS data, supplements to the NHIS have been conducted annually for the past 20 years.

The NHIS Supplement on Aging

One of the NHIS supplements is the Supplement on Aging. Conducted in 1984, it is a major source of information on long-term care services used by the elderly—particularly when used in conjunction with data collected by the Longitudinal Study on Aging, described below. Its purpose was to collect health and community service utilization information on the portion of the 1984 NHIS sample that was age 55 and over, which could be related back to the information regularly collected in the NHIS on these respondents. The SOA was administered to half the persons in the NHIS sample who were age 55-64 at the time of the interview and to all of those then age 65 and over.

The Longitudinal Study on Aging

The SOA is also the base for the Longitudinal Study of Aging, a prospective study of the same panel interviewed for the SOA. All respondents will be followed for at least six years by linkage with death records through the National Death Index. Respondents age 65 and over will be followed for at least six years by linkage with Medicare records. Those age 70 and over will be reinterviewed by telephone. The LSOA, which is based on a sample selected in 1984, provides extensive data on the health and medical history of a single cohort of the elderly.

Rapid changes in health, medical care needs, living arrangements, and available support are characteristic of the older population. The environment in which these personal changes occur is also in a constant state of flux. In order to understand the changing health needs of the older population, a sample should be selected from a new cohort and should be followed for at least five years— a plan that would permit measurement of some of the transitions occurring in the elderly population.

> **Recommendation 3.1:**   The panel recommends that the National Health Interview Survey's supplement on aging for the noninstitutionalized population ages 55 and over be repeated every 5 years. The sample should be followed for at least 5 years, and preferably 10 years, and interviewed for characteristics relevant to the older population as well as for changes in these characteristics.

The follow-up could be carried out by a combination of telephone calls and personal interviews with varying frequencies appropriate to the age of the sample member.

The Integrated System of Health Interview Surveys

The NCHS plans to replace the NHIS by 1989 with an Integrated System of Health Interview Surveys (ISHIS), which, although structurally different, will retain many of the attributes of the NHIS. It should still be possible to implement the panel's recommendations with the modified structure of the NHIS. The modification provides for core questions, the ability to link with other data bases, and surveys of special topics. The sample design consists of four panels, each a national probability sample of households. Core questions will be addressed to all four panels, although core items may be rotated from year to year. Emphasis is placed on the use of screening questions in the core to identify special subgroups of the population, e.g., veterans, who might then be followed in a special topic survey. The modifications also recognize the importance of being able to link

NHIS data with other data bases. The National Death Index will be checked routinely for all surveys to ascertain year and cause of death. Discussions are under way with the Health Care Financing Administration concerning the possibility of a follow-on survey of ISHIS participants to obtain their Medicare history. Provision will be made to explore special topics of current policy relevance, on request, with one or more of the panels. These special topic surveys will be funded externally.

The National Health and Nutrition Examination Surveys

The National Health and Nutrition Examination Surveys were established to collect those kinds of health data optimally obtained by direct physical examinations and physiological and biochemical measurements. The surveys measure the health and nutritional status of the U.S. population and permit estimation of the prevalence of certain diseases and the distributions of a broad variety of health-related measurements. NHANES I was conducted from 1971 to 1975; NHANES II was conducted from 1976 to 1980; current plans are under way for NHANES III to be fielded in 1988.

NHANES I and NHANES II did not include persons age 75 and over because it was anticipated that the logistics of bringing the frail elderly to the examination site would present serious problems, and any attempt to do so would result in a poor response rate. The growth of the older population has made it extremely important that this group be included in NHANES III. Ways must be found to make it possible to examine elderly people in their homes both to improve the response rate and to avoid the bias inherent in sampling only those able to come to the examination site.

Recommendation 3.2: The panel recommends that the National Institute on Aging and the National Center for Health Statistics support methodological work to increase the participation of older people in examination and interview surveys.

Recommendation 3.3: The panel recommends that the sample for NHANES III should not have an age cutoff. The panel further recommends that the sample of persons age 65 and over be adequate to provide suitably precise estimates of the prevalence of specific medical conditions among those over age 65.

The precision required in estimates depends on the planned analysis and therefore cannot be specified by the panel. When the precision desired in the estimates has been specified, computation of the required sample size is straightforward.[1]

Although NHANES I and II included questions on cognitive impairment, a more comprehensive set of measures for cognitive functioning and mental health should be included in NHANES III.

Recommendation 3.4: The panel recommends that the National Institute of Mental Health continue its development of diagnostic instruments for specific psychiatric disorders of major public health importance (e.g., schizophrenia, major depressions, and anxiety disorders as well as for cognitive impairments) that can be utilized in national health surveys, such as the NHIS and NHANES. The instrument should be added to the other medical assessment procedures utilized in these surveys.

The NHANES I Epidemiologic Follow-up Survey

The NHANES I Epidemiologic Follow-up Survey was first fielded in 1982-1984. The survey covered 14,407 persons who were ages 25-74 at the time they were examined in NHANES I, about 10 years

---

[1]The effective estimation of distributions of characteristics for the elderly and important subgroups of elderly (such as the 65-74, 75-84, and 85 and over age ranges) requires sufficient sample size. Such sample size is necessary in order for estimates to have sufficient precision to provide a meaningful description of these distributions. For attributes that apply to 20 to 80 percent of a subpopulation, a reasonable upper bound for the length of 95 percent confidence intervals from sample estimation is 10 percent. The minimum sample size required for this purpose is approximately n = 400. When the likelihood of an attribute is 10 to 20 percent (or 80 to 90 percent), narrower confidence intervals are needed so as to clearly indicate the extent to which estimates are bounded away from 0 percent (or 100 percent). As a result, a reasonable upper bound for the length of 95 percent confidence intervals in this setting is 6 percent, for which the minimum sample size needs to be n = 700. Even larger sample sizes are required for characteristics with likelihoods less than 10 percent (or greater than 90 percent).

Two other considerations also are relevant to sample size. One is whether the survey design involves clustering or other components that tend to lead to greater sampling variability than simple random sampling. The other is the extent to which the sample needs to provide a basis with suitable statistical power for comparisons among subgroups. Each of these considerations can lead to a doubling or larger increase in the previously discussed sample sizes.

before the follow-up visits; thus it included some persons in their eighties, but it did not reach the entire elderly population. The survey identified chronic disease risk factors associated with morbidity and mortality, ascertained changes in risk factors, morbidity, functional limitation, and institutionalization between NHANES I and the follow-up recontacts, and provided information to map the natural history of chronic diseases and functional impairments in the aging population. Continued follow-up of the elderly in the cohort was carried out in 1986 and of the entire cohort in 1987. It would be desirable to repeat the study following the NHANES III survey, particularly if it is expanded to reach the total elderly population. A longitudinal study for at least 10 years could produce useful information on changes in clinical assessments and laboratory measurements. Attrition in a follow-up survey may be very rapid among the very old. With an oversample of the older ages in NHANES III, a 2-year cycle for resurvey might be feasible and productive of measures of change.

> **Recommendation 3.5:** The panel recommends that a follow-up study to NHANES III be carried out that is expanded to reach the older age groups and provides for repeated observations, preferably at 2-year intervals but at a maximum interval of 5 years.

Data on Cause of Death

To ascertain which nonrespondents have died in a longitudinal survey of the health status of the elderly, it is essential to match nonrespondents against the National Death Index (NDI), unless there are other definitive ways of identifying deaths. Social Security number is a key item of information in such a survey, since it is needed for matching with the NDI. Once a death record has been found in the NDI, information on the cause of death can be obtained from the appropriate state health department.

Obviously, the NDI can also be used to obtain information on date and cause of death for sample members in any survey, whether cross-sectional or longitudinal. Consistent follow-up with the NDI for sample members age 55 and over in surveys that collect data on health status could lead to an extremely rich repository of information for relating health status at one or more points in life to age at and cause of death. NCHS has provided for such follow-up with the NDI in the long-range plans for the Integrated System of Health Interview Surveys.

> **Recommendation 3.6:**   The panel recommends that sample populations age 55 or over in all health-related surveys of individuals be followed by matching with the National Death Index to identify deaths and subsequently obtaining cause of death information from state health departments. All health-related surveys should include the respondent's Social Security number.

The Importance of Longitudinal Studies

Longitudinal data sets are increasingly important for two reasons. The first is to provide dynamic descriptions of aging as a process rather than static descriptions of elderly people at a particular historical moment. Aging is a continuous process, beginning at birth and ending at death. To understand that process, to identify and trace the pathways that individuals take through the successive years requires longitudinal data. Inferences drawn by comparing people in different age groups rather than following individuals through the aging process are often tentative and subject to significant restrictions in interpretation.

In the later years of life, longitudinal data track the movement of individuals through the stages of morbidity, disability, and mortality. When coupled with measurement of specific endpoints, including dysfunction, disability, overt disease states, development of cognitive dysfunction, and cognitive competence, such data sets might provide insight into the transition points in the development of frailty. Longitudinal data sets can also take into account the latency that characterizes the development of chronic diseases, the often long period between the recognition of a disease and its functional impact. Longitudinal data sets provide the capacity to establish patterns of change over time in individuals, which is increasingly important with the recognition of the tremendous variability among the elderly.

A second reason for requiring longitudinal data on the aging process relates to causal inference. Static data can show, for example, the characteristics of men and women who are aging successfully, but they cannot show us which, if any, of those characteristics are causes of their success. Tentative inferences can be made from longitudinal data (which pin down temporal order) and then tested by experimental efforts to decrease morbidity and mortality and increase productive and satisfying life.

The increasing geriatric population has stimulated interest in research in all aspects of care of the elderly. The field is changing rapidly as these efforts yield new information regarding disease prevention, early detection of treatable causes of disability, and successful management of these disorders. Recognition of the special characteristics of the elderly will guide collection of data, permitting further advances in understanding the interaction of normal aging and disease, the factors underlying the variability among the elderly, and the important health transitions they experience in the later years of life.

To understand the illness histories of the elderly, recording the health status and lifestyle of these individuals earlier in life becomes important for many reasons. Among them are the association of psychological factors in middle age with morbidity later in life, the effects of risk-enhancing behavior in middle age on subsequent morbidity, and the need to identify the transition points from one functional status or health state to another. It is also important to track people who have certain diagnoses, such as high blood pressure, from an early point to see the functional consequences at later points in time; or to identify 55-year-olds who have a diagnosis of diabetes to see what functional losses accompany that early diagnosis and what the distribution of impairment is in that subpopulation at some later point in time. For these reasons longitudinal studies should start before age 65. Although there is no uniform age at which it is ideal to start tracking transitions in health that affect the elderly, for practical reasons as well as the fact that changes appear to concentrate in the decade prior to age 65, age 55 is a desirable starting point for many longitudinal studies.

Recommendation 3.7: The panel recommends that all surveys designed to study the health status of the elderly, particularly longitudinal surveys, start at age 55 and have the capacity to provide information for five-year age groups.

Even though there have been cohort studies in the past, studies with new cohorts are needed because of possible cohort differences. A cohort age 55 in 1966 may differ in important ways from a cohort of that age in 1986. The period of life between age 55 and 70 is a critical transition period that warrants current study. In summary, longitudinal studies can help address one of the major data gaps in the health status area—the elucidation of the illness histories of the elderly—by providing data to serve the following purposes:

(1) clarify the relation between the presence of disease states (e.g., diagnosis of cancer, hypertension, diabetes) and the subsequent progressive emergence of symptoms of illness, functional impairment, and eventual mortality.

(2) determine what kinds of individuals are more susceptible to a disease process;

(3) focus on the factors influencing the transition from one health state to another;

(4) determine the relation between improved longevity and changes in morbidity (i.e., compression of morbidity);

(5) recognize that health status can improve or deteriorate over time and measure the extent of changes in both directions in tracing an illness history;

(6) identify the multiple potential pathways that individuals might take through the various stages of illness.

FUNCTIONAL STATUS

Health survey data show a pattern in which vigorous old age predominates. Most older Americans live in the community and are cognitively intact and fully independent in their activities of daily living (Rowe, 1985). Dependency and institutionalization are the exception. However, major functional impairment is clearly age-related among the elderly; approximately 5 percent of individuals ages 65-74 require assistance in basic activities of daily living, while 35 percent require such assistance by age 85 (National Center for Health Statistics, 1983a).

"Even if one maintains functional independence into old age, the risk of becoming frail for a long period is still high" (Rowe, 1985:828). One study (Katz et al., 1983) found that for independent persons between the ages of 65 and 69, "active life expectancy"— that portion of the remaining years characterized by independence— represents about 60 percent of total life expectancy; by age 85, that portion falls to 40 percent (see Figure 3.1; see also Figure 4.1).

Characteristics of Functional Status

"Health is a state of complete physical, mental, and social well-being and not merely the absence of disease or infirmity" (World

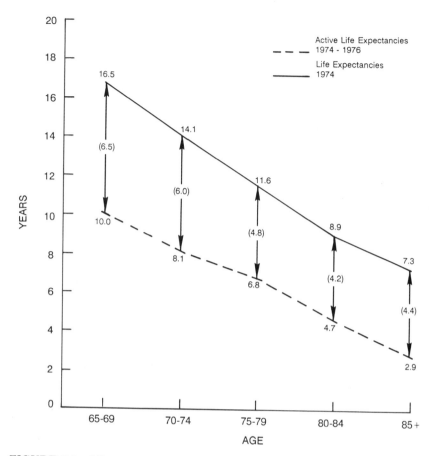

FIGURE 3.1   Life expectancies and active life expectancies in Massachusetts.

Health Organization, 1948). Although well-known, this definition has not been applied to produce measures of well-being. The familiar measures of health are generally measures of illness, and, for the elderly, measures of the need for assistance. Measures of the functional status of the active elderly are needed to trace the transitions from their well state to states of disability along the continuum of health.

Most of the well-known measures describe functional status along one of four dimensions: physical function, cognitive function, mental health function, and social function. Some gerontologists add a fifth dimension, economic status, to these areas of measurement.

Physical Function

Physical function scales are of two types: self-reported and performance tests. The self-reported tests vary in the limitations they measure among the active elderly as contrasted with the elderly needing care. For example, one scale (the original or adaptation of the Katz Activities of Daily Living—ADL—Index) typically identifies approximately 10 percent of the noninstitutionalized elderly population with limitations (Katz et al., 1983). A second scale (an adaptation of the Rosow-Breslau Functional Health Scale) typically identifies approximately 40 percent of the well elderly who report limitations in one of three areas: the ability to walk a half mile, to climb stairs, to do heavy housework (Rosow and Breslau, 1966). The third common scale, based on items developed by Nagi (1976) for the Social Security Disability Surveys, typically identifies approximately 70 percent of the elderly who are living in the community as reporting difficulty in performing one or more activities such as stooping, crouching, kneeling, fingering small objects, extending arms above shoulder level, pushing or pulling large objects, and lifting weights above 10 pounds.

Performance tests of physical function include a 15-minute manual dexterity performance test described by Williams et al. (1982), a hand grasp performance test, a pulmonary function test, and blood pressure measurements (both standing and seated). Actual performance of some of the tasks on the ADL scale has been part of the examinations in the Framingham study.

Cognitive Function

In tests of cognitive function, performance tests are used more frequently than self-reported measures. Among the performance tests frequently used in community surveys of older people are a variety of tests (e.g., the Mini-Mental Scale Examination in the Epidemiologic Catchment Area Project) that are intended to measure orientation to time and place. In addition, community surveys often use subscales from intelligence tests and other sources to gauge short-term and long-term memory and certain other cognitive capacities.

The self-reported tests of cognitive function include items asking the respondent's judgment of his or her memory capacity at present compared with specified earlier intervals.

Mental Health Function

In the measurement of mental function, self-reported assessments are used almost exclusively in this country, where epidemiologic studies are generally performed by lay interviewers. In contrast, clinicians have been involved in studies in Europe, and have therefore made psychiatric diagnoses as traditionally done in a clinician's office. Our understanding of some aspects of mental functioning would be enhanced through the combination of screening procedures and standardized diagnostic interviews. Standardized measures of morale and depression that can be used in community surveys are: the Lawton Morale Scale, the Center for Epidemiological Studies-Depression Scale (CES-D) (Radloff, 1977) designed by the National Institute of Mental Health (NIMH), and the Beck Depression Scale, among others. In addition, NIMH has sponsored the development and field testing of the Diagnostic Interview Schedule (DIS), which approximates the DSMIII (Diagnostic and Statistical Manual, 3d edition) categorization of clinical diagnoses and can be administered by lay interviewers. The DIS was developed for use in the Epidemiological Catchment Area Projects.

Social Function

For measuring social function, numerous self-reported items are used in community surveys. The Alameda County Study (Berkman and Breslow, 1983) and the National Institute on Aging's Established Populations for Epidemiologic Studies of the Elderly project (Cornoni-Huntley et al., 1986) are two examples.

Assessing Functional Status

There are numerous functional tests in addition to those discussed above. Several recent studies have listed and described the existing tests (Kane and Kane, 1981; Mangen and Peterson, 1982; Fillenbaum, 1984). In her study published by the World Health Organization (WHO) in 1984, Fillenbaum argues for a multidimensional approach to functional status (p.5):

> There have been few attempts to make a comprehensive assessment of the well-being of representative groups of elderly people as a basis for policy decisions concerning the provision of appropriate services. Rather than considering the elderly person as an integral human being, the tendency of care givers and research

workers alike has been to measure single dimensions of well-being, such as mental function, social support, economic status, physical morbidity, or capacity for self-care. However, elderly people are subject to multiple disadvantages, and their physical, mental, social, and economic well-being are closely interrelated—more so than at younger ages—so that combined assessment of the various dimensions of well-being is necessary.

There is a general consensus that five basic dimensions should be included in any overall assessment of elderly individuals within a population, namely activities of daily living, mental health, physical health, and social and economic functioning. While it is necessary and important to have information on specific areas, functioning in one area has an impact on functioning in others. Assessment not only should be multidimensional, but also should be in terms of functional status.

Fillenbaum focuses on three multidimensional functional assessments: the comprehensive assessment and referral evaluation (CARE), the Philadelphia Geriatric Center multilevel assessment instrument (MAI), and the Older American Resources and Services multidimensional functional assessment questionnaire—selected because they meet standards of validity and reliability. In addition, Fillenbaum also describes the Rand Health Insurance Study (RAND HIS) questionnaire. While it was designed for use at ages below 61, the original questionnaire was actually used in the Rand study with persons up to age 85. With minor alterations this questionnaire could be made fully relevant to an older population.

Fillenbaum also notes the existence of the International Classification of Impairments, Disabilities, and Handicaps (ICIDH), which can be used in the classification of handicaps on a 10-point scale, with 0 indicating the absence of a handicap. The classification was published by WHO in 1980, but it has not been used in the United States. It should be reviewed for possible use of those parts of the classification that could be adapted to descriptions of the well elderly.

The U.S. Social Security Administration's Longitudinal Retirement History Survey (SSA LRHS) is cited as an example of the use of a multidimensional functional questionnaire over a long period—6 years. To illustrate the utility of such survey results, Fillenbaum uses data from the SSA LRHS to develop a transition matrix showing the estimated transition probabilities from each 1969 health state to each 1971 state for the LRHS sample (Fillenbaum, 1984:62). Each of the five dimensions is treated as a bivariate (impaired or not impaired) yielding a matrix with 32 rows and 32 columns.

There is a need to reexamine existing tests and questionnaires for use in surveys of the general population of the elderly and to develop new instruments if needed. One criterion for determining the suitability of an instrument is its capacity to provide information for measuring the complete spectrum of health from well-being to illness and dependency and the transition rates from one state to another over time. The second criterion for selection should be the feasibility of applying the questionnaire in an interview survey. The third criterion should be whether the instrument is sufficiently brief for use in national information systems.

Recommendation 3.8: The panel recommends (a) that the National Center for Health Services Research and Health Care Technology Assessment, the National Institute of Mental Health, and the National Institute on Aging support research to develop, enhance, and evaluate instruments for measuring functional status (physical, mental health, cognitive, and social) based on the behavior of active older people; (b) that the National Center for Health Statistics continue and enhance its effort to determine how well these instruments address the health status of the elderly and how the instruments might be adapted (reduced) for application in national information systems; and (c) that the National Institute on Aging and the National Center for Health Statistics support methodological work to improve the validity and reliability of measures of cognitive and physical impairments of the elderly.

The emphasis in the provision of health care to the elderly should be on maintaining functional capability and increasing active life expectancy. Evaluation of the elderly patient must focus on what the patient can do, relative to what the patient should be able or wishes to do, and on identification of recent functional deficits that may be reversible. Although a complete and precise diagnosis is essential, the functional impact of each diagnosis should be evaluated. Functional measures should include not only activities of daily living (bathing, continence, dressing, eating, mobility, and walking) and instrumental activities of daily living (e.g., doing housework/laundry, preparing meals, shopping, getting around outside, going places not within walking distance, managing money, taking medicines, using the telephone) but also more subtle effects of disease on cognitive functions. Specific diagnoses often have little relation to functional status and the length of the diagnosis list provides little insight into the specific needs and capabilities of a particular patient. Too often a long diagnosis list biases physicians to think that the patient is multiply impaired and therefore frail, although this may not be the case at all. Diagnoses themselves are often a weak criterion for assessing the health care needs of the elderly (Besdine, 1983).

QUALITY OF LIFE

The General Concept

Several of the topics discussed earlier in this chapter are related to the quality of life, which for older persons includes the extension of longevity, the compression of morbidity, health and functional status, and psychosocial factors as modifiers of disease. This section discusses some of the components of quality of life, including measures of productive activity of the elderly, and shows their relationship to those topics.

Age is not a strong predictor of subjective well-being. By and large, older people are no less satisfied with their lives than those who are young. Indeed, when one looks at satisfaction with the various life domains—income and standard of living, work, family and marriage, friendships, housing and community, leisure, and health itself—only satisfaction with health declines with age. In other words, people tend to come to terms with their lives, and most people do not experience the terms as unduly harsh (Herzog et al., 1982).

For persons of all ages, including the elderly, the quality of life experienced by an individual is related to his or her level of satisfaction with life, sense of well-being, and feeling of self-worth and self-esteem (Campbell et al., 1976; Andrews and Withey, 1976). In contrast to objective social indicators for the population or particular subgroups, which focus on socially significant observable events or characteristics (such as marital status and employment), quality-of-life measures are concerned with the subjective, psychological experiences that surround or accompany these events or characteristics, as perceived and reported by the individual (such as the level of pride and satisfaction derived from employment). Correlations between objective social indicators and perceived quality of life for an individual tend to be weak (Vinokur et al., 1983:32).

Level of satisfaction has been measured globally, referring to overall satisfaction with life; with respect to domains of life experience, such as health and mental health, marriage, family life, friendships, housing, job or work, nonwork and leisure activities, and financial situation (personal assets, financial security, earnings); and on such dimensions as personal safety and the security of one's possessions (the latter for institutionalized persons in particular) (see, e.g., Campbell et al., 1976; Gastil, 1978; George and Bearon, 1980; Morgan and Smith, 1969). This view of quality of life presupposes that an individual has aspirations and expectations that serve as the criterion or standard against which his or her current situation is perceived and assessed. The level of congruence between expectations and perceived or actual circumstances is viewed as generating a subjective evaluation of satisfaction or dissatisfaction, which is for that individual a measure or indicator of quality of life, either globally or for the particular domain in question (Franklin et al., 1984).

Personal well-being, also a contributor to one's perceived quality of life, is a broader concept than satisfaction with life or its domains. According to its proponents (including Bharadwaj and Wilkening, 1977, 1980), this notion involves self-development, the realization of one's own potential as an individual and as a social being (deriving from Maslow, 1954), and the capacity to adapt to change and is equivalent to a sense of personal efficacy (Vinokur et al., 1983:34).

Feelings of self-worth and self-esteem are also related to a person's assessment of the quality of his or her life (see George and Bearon, 1980). The belief that one's achievements and activities are valued and needed by others and the perception that one is capable of interacting and negotiating successfully with the environment enhance feelings of self-worth and self-esteem.

Some Dimensions of Quality of Life

Health Status

While health status is only one among many dimensions that affect a person's assessment of the quality of his or her life, it is a very important one. George and Bearon (1980), for example, regard general health (and functional) status as one of four dimensions that define quality of life for older persons, along with socioeconomic status, general life satisfaction, and self-esteem and related measures. As defined here, health status consists of physical, psychological, and social components. The focus of survey questionnaires is typically on physical symptoms and the functioning of organs and systems, the ability to perform life roles, and the ability to move about. Measures of psychological health focus on psychological symptoms and disorders. Social health is most often defined in terms of an individual's ability to function as a member of the community, including the world of work, and involves the nature of family relationships, friendships, and community participation (Vinokur et al., 1983). Yet here, as for the other domains of life, subjective estimates of one's physical health and well-being do not necessarily correlate with objective measures based on laboratory findings and physical examinations (Vinokur et al., 1983). That is, the relationship between the presence of actual disease and disability and perceived well-being is neither obvious nor uniform across medical conditions. Similarly, neither increased life expectancy nor the use of medical interventions that objectively improve medical conditions invariably results in the perception that one's quality of life has been improved (Vinokur et al., 1983).

Satisfaction with Life

The elderly tend to be as globally satisfied with their lives, on the whole, as younger persons, though their level of satisfaction with their health status tends to decline as they advance in years. They also tend to report their health as good or excellent and to see themselves as functioning well. Lengthening of the life span—or longevity—per se will not result in enhanced satisfaction with life for the elderly unless personal vigor and the ability to function independently (without institutionalization) are maintained. As noted above, it is not known yet whether increased life expectancy will be accompanied by an overall increase in active life expectancy for the elderly, or rather by a prolongation of the period of dependency and functional impairment, which does tend to increase with age. In this connection, it is worth reiterating that aging does not inevitably result in decline of health status or function: older persons are very heterogeneous with respect to health and functional status, and improvement in both—successful aging—can and does occur.

Functional Status

Functional status—including the ability to perform self-care activities and to carry out activities of daily living such as cooking, shopping, and cleaning—is more critical to quality of life than morbidity or diagnosis per se. Physical, cognitive, mental health, and social functioning, individually and together, as they tend to reinforce each other, contribute to a sense of well-being and satisfaction with life.

Availability of Social Support System

The availability of a social support system, including actual and potential informal supports such as family and friends, is crucial to the quality of life for the elderly, whether residing in the community or in an institution. Not only are positive, close, and stable family relationships correlated with satisfaction with life (see, for example, Najman and Levine, 1981), but also the availability of social supports can prevent or delay institutionalization of frail elderly people.

Productive Activity

Increasing longevity should be accompanied not only by the maintenance or enhancement of physical, mental health, emotional, and social function, but also by productive activity that is recognized by oneself and others as socially useful.

The development of statistics on the full range of productive activities, especially among older men and women, is important for both scientific reasons and national policy. Both require the broadening of national statistical series so that they represent more accurately the major activity patterns of men and women throughout the life course. The lengthening of life, if it is to be meaningful to individuals and enriching rather than burdensome to the society as a whole, must be made as productive as possible. Measurement of the extent to which this goal is achieved, requires accurate statistics on the current productivity of older people and statistical information on the factors that determine that productivity.

National data of this kind are not now available. Instead, all paid employment is assumed to be productive and all unpaid contributions to society (except for work on a family farm or business) are ignored. These omissions are especially problematic for policy purposes because they are age-biased. They not only underestimate productive activity in the nation as a whole; they differentially underestimate the productive contributions of different age and gender groups.

The underestimation is greatest for those past the usual age of retirement. When people leave paid employment, they drop from the conventional statistics of productive behavior—for example, the Current Population Survey no longer counts them as "in the labor force" and consequently they are also omitted from statistics derived from the CPS, for example, the gross national product (GNP). People, including the elderly, who are homemakers, who care for ill or disabled family members, who do volunteer work in schools or hospitals are classified as nonworkers—as recipients and consumers who do not produce. Policy debates over compulsory retirement, pension entitlements, Social Security funding, and the like are therefore conducted with only a partial base of knowledge, since they do not take cognizance of the important productive work of the elderly.

The development of more comprehensive measures of productive behavior must begin with a conceptual task: the definition of activities that are to be defined as productive. We propose a definition that is primarily economic: an activity is productive if it generates valued goods or services, and the key measure of its productivity is the market value (actual or attributed) of those goods and services minus the nonlabor costs involved in their production.

Several properties of productive behavior follow from this definition:

(1) With the exception of paid employment, for which the market value is established by the payment, no other activity is currently counted as productive; market value must be estimated or attributed for these activities under the proposed definition.

(2) Paid employment includes work done in both the regular and irregular (reported and unreported) economies. It thus includes untaxed and typically unreported payment received for work, as well as pay or profit from regular employment.

(3) Unpaid activities that generate goods or services, and for which market values can be determined, are likely to include housework, child care, care of ill or disabled family members or friends, and some forms of volunteer work in organizations. For example, the activities of a volunteer who types letters or does bookkeeping for a civic organization fall within our definition; mere attendance at the meetings of the organization would not.

(4) The proposed definition permits the inclusion of activities in which the producer is also the consumer of the product,

provided that such activities generate goods or services for which a clear market value can be attributed.

As an example of the implications of this approach, consider the painting of a house, an activity that might be undertaken by a professional painter for wages on a regular job or as a contract for profit. The same activity, however, might be undertaken for pay by a person working outside a regular job. It might also be done by a relative or friend without pay of any kind and, finally, it might be done by the homeowner himself or herself.

The definitions and procedures of current government statistics would include the first of these—house painting done as part of a regular job for pay or profit—in its measures of employment, and ultimately, its contribution to GNP. The second case—house painting done as part of the irregular economy—might or might not be included. The third variation, in which the work is done as a favor to a relative or friend, would not be included. And the fourth case, in which the same work is done by a person for himself or herself, would certainly not be included. Yet in all these cases, the work done is identical. Ultimately, such work should be included in our national statistics in such a way that it would be possible to distinguish between paid and unpaid work, and between work done for others and that done for oneself.

Recommendation 3.9: The panel recommends that the Department of Labor, in conjunction with the Bureau of the Census and the Department of Health and Human Services, develop a concept of productive activity that includes both paid and unpaid work and that can be measured and reported in surveys such as the Current Population Survey, the National Health Interview Survey, and the Survey of Income and Program Participation, as well as in the decennial census.

Implementation of this recommendation would recognize the fact that longer life means, for many elderly people, increased productive years that have the potential to contribute to an individual's sense of self-esteem and self-worth and thereby enhance his or her quality of life. Once the concept of productive activity that includes both paid and unpaid work has been developed and made operational for purposes of collecting data via surveys, the quality of the productive life of the elderly should be monitored.

In the absence of such statistics, no authoritative measures of these categories of unpaid work are available, but estimates have been made (Goldschmidt-Clermont, 1982; Peskin, 1983). They differ, but all of them indicate that the goods and services generated by unpaid work are substantial relative to conventionally estimated monetary GNP. No estimates of unpaid work set its total value as less than 20 percent of GNP, and some estimates range as high as 44 percent of GNP.

Some development of measures has been done on all of the broad activity categories with which we are concerned: paid employment, unpaid voluntary work in organizational and informal settings, and work that produces goods for one's own consumption. All of these available measures involve self-report to some extent. For example, unpaid work to operate a family farm or business is measured by the Bureau of the Census in comparable terms—number of hours worked, occupation, and industry—to those for paid employment. Other forms of unpaid work, either in organizational settings or on less formal bases, have been measured less frequently, less success-fully, and less completely. The Current Population Survey provides estimates of the number of people who are engaged in housework and are not working for pay or profit. Mutual assistance of various kinds has been measured mainly in terms of frequency of contact and self-rated importance of the relations involved. The CPS incorpo-rates no estimates of the monetary value of such work, but reviews of alternative methods for making such estimates are available (see, e.g., Goldschmidt-Clermont, 1982; Peskin, 1983).

Measures of self-care have been developed, with scales of physi-cal self-maintenance and daily living (Lawton, 1977; Kane and Kane, 1981). The full range of activities in which the individual consumes the product of his or her own work, however, has not been systemat-ically measured.

Given the state of measurement development and the goal of assessing the full range of productive activities throughout the life course, the panel proposes five sets of measures: (1) categories of productive activity engaged in, (2) amount of input (hours devoted) to such activities, (2) monetary value of the product or service result-ing from each of these activity categories on an individual basis, (4) self-evaluation of the productivity of the activity, and (5) outcomes for the individual engaging in the activity and for others. These suggestions are based on a set of propositions for which substan-tial evidence is already available: that the reality and experience of producing something of value or of providing a service and the of producing something of value or of providing a service and the recognition and acknowledgment of that fact by oneself and others are conducive to improving quality of life.

Quality of Life for the Institutionalized Elderly

For older persons who reside in institutions such as nursing homes rather than in the community, the factors that contribute to satisfaction with life, a sense of well-being, and feelings of self-worth are somewhat different from those discussed above. Already limited in their health status and ability to function independently and autonomously in the community—two contributors to a high quality of life—such persons perceive their quality of life as heavily dependent on the quality of their medical and nursing care. This is especially true for the very ill and disabled (Institute of Medicine, 1986). A recent empirical study shows that nursing home residents also attach high importance to the qualifications, competence, and attitudes of staff—particularly nurse's aides who provide much of the hands-on care on a day-to-day basis. Friendliness, cheerfulness, and the treatment of residents with respect and dignity are qualities highly valued in staff and are viewed as contributing heavily to residents' quality of life (Institute of Medicine, 1986). In addition, such amenities as the quality of the food, the ambiance, the ability to make personal choices and participate in planning one's own care, and activities that assist residents in maintaining or regaining independent function (such as rehabilitation exercises, encouragement in ambulation or self-feeding) contribute to a high quality of life for the institutionalized elderly (Institute of Medicine, 1986).

Conclusion

In order to document the quality of life experienced by older persons, both community residents and those residing in institutions, new measures, suitable for cross-sectional and longitudinal surveys, will have to be developed.

Recommendation 3.10: The panel recommends that national population-based surveys such as the National Health Interview Survey and the National Nursing Home Survey (which includes a population component) include measures of factors that influence quality of life both positively and negatively as people progress to advanced ages.

4
Health Transitions and the Compression of Morbidity

Public policy debates in the areas of health and medical care have emerged in recent years around the question of whether improvements in lifestyle and medical technology will delay the onset of chronic illness and disability and result in a compression of morbidity at older ages. If the incidence of chronic illness declines and morbidity is compressed to a very brief period at the end of the life span, there will be a growing number of healthy people at the older ages. One set of policy issues emerges from this scenario:

- What is the appropriate age for retirement?
- Will a relatively smaller working population be able to pay Social Security payroll taxes for the growing number and proportion of the retired elderly?
- Can productive employment be found for the growing number of healthy older persons in the face of relatively high and persistent unemployment?
- What is the viability of tax credits, reverse mortgages, independent retirement accounts (IRAs), and other saving plans in assisting the future elderly to pay for a greater share of their future health and long-term care costs?
- Will income maintenance and social welfare programs be adequate to meet the needs of the elderly with longer life expectancy?

Under another scenario relating to the compression of morbidity, improvements in survival may postpone chronic illness and disability to older ages, raising a different set of policy questions:

- Will medical and social services be available to maintain the independence at home of the growing number of chronically ill and functionally disabled elderly people, avoiding institutionalization?
- Can we develop various types of supportive living arrangements for the growing number of women age 75 and older with no spouse who live alone?
- Will public and private income support and medical care programs be adequate to meet the needs of the growing number of disabled persons?
- What type of rehabilitative programs should be designed and made available for physically impaired elderly populations?

In assessing health transitions in old and very old populations, a number of conceptual, measurement, and analytic issues emerge that are not as evident in younger populations. These issues emerge for a number of reasons.

First, and perhaps most important, is the different nature of disease, disease interactions, and physiology in older persons. These concerns focus on the nature of intraindividual changes in health at later ages. There are numerous age-related changes in the physiological state of the individual, for example, changes in metabolism, immune response, and organ function, a greater likelihood of accumulating significant adverse environmental exposures, and the cumulative effects of multiple chronic conditions and diseases. Intraindividual changes in health at later ages involve these age-related changes and the effect of such changes on the manifestations of specific disease processes.

Intrinsic to these concerns is the fact that the chronic diseases and conditions tend to manifest a different time scale than acute disease processes more typical at younger ages. In particular, the period of time over which chronic diseases become manifest in the elderly tends to become significant with respect to the total life span and to the amount of life expectancy at later ages. This greater period of time means that, even if the incidence rates of chronic disease were unchanged with age, there would be a greater probability that older individuals would accumulate multiple diseases, and the time over which the older person would have these multiple (and interacting) diseases simultaneously would be longer. Even if such chronic diseases become manifest at younger ages, the physiological reserves to preserve homeostasis are generally stronger at those ages, and the duration of disease expression may be shorter with disease control (if not cure) more completely and rapidly imposed by the physiology of younger persons. Alternatively, if a chronic disease is atypically manifest at younger ages, it may be due to particularly powerful genetic or other susceptibilities to these disease processes, in which case the natural course of the disease may be dramatically shortened by loss of homeostatic control and death.

Thus, health transitions at later ages cannot be described simply in terms of the incidence rate of independent disease events. Instead they must be viewed in terms of multiple, interacting disease processes that operate in a host with generally declining homeostatic reserve. It is clear that these concepts involve modeling health changes in the elderly person as changes in a complex multidimensional system evolving over a considerable period of time.

To do so requires addressing formidable measurement and analytic problems that are not well handled by our current data collection and analytic strategies. The practical need for such data and analytic strategies is already manifest by the underlying concepts in the development of clinical specialties in geriatric medicine (e.g., Minaker and Rowe, 1985; Besdine, 1984) and in concerns with the special problems in clinically managing and treating specific diseases (e.g., lung cancer, breast cancer, isolated systolic hypertension, diabetes) in older persons.

It should also be noted that there are many examples of such complex system-based models in the physical sciences that could be the point of departure for developing appropriate health transition models for the elderly. The development of such models, however, requires an approach or philosophy of inference that differs from the approach typically employed in experimental or clinical trial designs; that is, we wish to develop an approximate mathematical description of a complex physical system rather than to test whether an observed effect would have reasonably occurred simply by chance.

In addition to these differences in health states and their changes in elderly individuals, other issues emerge in modeling the health changes in the populations of the elderly. These arise because people who are alive at later ages represent only a portion of their cohorts, since significant mortality will have occurred in these cohorts— mortality that will systematically select out persons according to the health characteristics we wish to assess. Issues in measurement also occur because, though disease prevalence may increase, population prevalence (i.e., the number of persons available for study in any well-defined population) at very advanced ages is small. Furthermore, the description of the disease process becomes complex and the rate of changes in physiological state may accelerate when homeostatic mechanisms become weaker at advanced ages or due to the accumulation of multiple disease processes. This complexity of disease state may make even the development of crude indicators of health state at advanced ages more difficult (e.g., the need for multiple-cause mortality data rather than underlying-cause mortality data to describe mortality patterns among the oldest-old).

From the above discussion, it is clear that new concepts and models that are based on process and duration rather than on event and incidence need to be developed to assess health changes at later ages. Indeed, the many recent debates that have emerged in the biomedical and health policy literature about the direction of recent health changes at later ages may be due simply to the lack of common concepts and models. It is clear, however, that the complexity of the physical system being described makes it difficult to have a parsimonious and relatively simple conceptual model to help inform the debate and improve concepts and communication.

In order to remedy this problem, a World Health Organization Scientific Advisory Group (World Health Organization, 1984) developed a model of health transitions at later ages. This model is based on simple life-table concepts in order to develop a theoretical framework that would be readily understood at the policy level. The basic model is actually quite simple, as shown in Figure 4.1.

Figure 4.1 contains a series of three survival curves labeled mortality, disability, and morbidity. The outermost curve (mortality) represents the effects of mortality on overall survival. We see that the proportion surviving from a cohort to each successive age declines (i.e., as one progresses to the right on the horizontal axis). In addition to the overall survival curve, there are survival curves for chronic morbidity and chronic disability. The lowest survival curve (morbidity) represents the probability of surviving to a given age free of chronic morbidity. The area labeled A under this curve represents the number of person-years that a person in this cohort could expect to survive free of disease (i.e., healthy life expectancy).

The middle curve, labeled disability, describes the probability of surviving to a given age free of serious chronic disability. The formulation assumes that disability emerges as a result of the progression of some underlying morbid process. This curve identifies two additional areas in the figure.

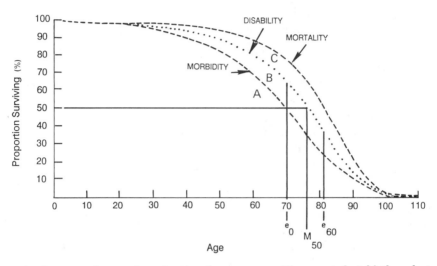

e_0 and e_{60} are the number of years of autonomous life expected at birth and at age 60, respectively. M_{50} is the age to which 50 percent of females could expect to survive without loss of autonomy.

FIGURE 4.1   The observed mortality and hypothetical morbidity and disability survival curves for females in the United States of America in 1980.

Source: World Health Organization (1984). Reprinted by permission.

The first, the area between the morbidity and disability survival curves labeled B, defines the number of person-years that can be expected to be lived by an individual from the cohort in a morbid, but disability-free, state. This portion of the figure has implications for acute health services, but relatively little direct impact on long-term care services. Many of the diseases that are fatal in middle age may produce a significant contribution to this portion of the figure— but relatively little to the disabled person-years to be experienced by the cohort. Examples of this type of disease process are cancer and myocardial infarctions.

The second area defined by the disability curve lies between it and the mortality curve and is labeled C. This area represents the person-years that can be expected to be lived by a person from this cohort in a chronically morbid and disabled state. Recall that the total area under the disability curve (areas A and B) represents the number of person-years that can be expected to be lived in a disability-free state. This total area may be viewed therefore as a measure of active or autonomous life expectancy (e.g., Koizumi, 1982; Katz et al., 1983; Wilkins and Adams, 1983). Certain disease processes will have a maximum effect on active life expectancy; for example, onset of a serious stroke or Alzheimer's disease may immediately produce serious disability. Such diseases have serious consequences for long-term care as well as acute care services.

With the three survival curves, it is possible to more precisely distinguish between the positions of different analysts about changes in health at advanced ages. For example, a major area of debate has centered on whether the health status of elderly persons has improved at each age as life expectancy at later ages increased. This debate was central to discussions about whether the entitlement age for social security could reasonably be increased from 65 to 67 to adjust for a two-year increase in life expectancy for males at age 65. Some analysts argued (e.g., Feldman, 1983) that life expectancy increased because chronically ill and morbid persons were surviving for longer periods of time. This could be represented in Figure 4.1 by the mortality survival curve moving to the right but the morbidity and disability curves remaining unchanged. This would increase the absolute numbers of years expected to be spent by a population in morbid and disabled states as well as the ratio of dependent morbid person-years of life to the total number of person-years expected to be lived.

The majority opinion was that as the mortality curve moved to the right, both the morbidity and disability curves moved to the right in a reasonably "parallel" fashion. Thus, the probability of surviving to age 67 free of disease and disability was the same after the recent life expectancy increases at later ages as it had been at age 65 before the increase. This suggests that the ratio of disabled and morbid person-years to be lived to the total would decline, raising the questions of how this improvement could be turned to society's benefit.

These discussions relate to a topic currently of considerable interest: the compression of morbidity. This concept suggests that different public health policies will have different effects on how rapidly each of the three curves moves to the right. For example, focusing exclusively on treating diseases after they emerge may cause life expectancy to increase but allow the age at onset of disease and disability to remain the same, with a net increase in the number of years lived in a morbid and disabled state. Alternatively, certain prevention and health promotion strategies may delay the age at onset of disease more than life expectancy is increased. In this case, the period spent in a morbid state and the acute health resources required may be reduced. Interestingly, recent data suggest that the diseases responsible for most of the disability and dependence at advanced ages (e.g., arthritis, Alzheimer's disease) are not those typically targeted by prevention efforts (e.g., heart disease and cancer). Thus, without careful attention to the effects of prevention on disability as well as disease, the morbid period may be decreased (decreasing acute health care costs) but the disabled period might be relatively untouched—thus having little effect on aggregate needs for long-term care (Manton, 1986b). Alternatively, the rate of progress of the disease may be retarded so that the age at onset of disability may increase more than life expectancy. In this case, the disabled period is compressed or reduced.

A specific example of the effects of such compression was discussed by Brody (1987). He points out that the risk of hip fracture increases roughly exponentially with age. As a consequence, if the age at onset curve of hip fracture could be shifted five years to the right (i.e., the process retarded five years, perhaps by nutritional supplementation or hormonal therapy), the prevalence of hip fracture in the population would be cut in half, provided there were no corresponding increases in life expectancy.

One extreme form of the compression of morbidity argument (Fries, 1980, 1983) suggests that the United States and other developed countries currently have life expectancies near to their biological limits. As a consequence, the survival curve for mortality will have little potential to move much to the right with a corresponding rapid increase in the prevalence of death due to biological senescence, i.e., natural death (Fries, 1983). Since natural death is argued to be due to senescent processes, it is also argued that it will be independent of the chronic disease processes that produce disability. Thus, while the mortality curve is fixed, the age at onset of disease and disability can be delayed by appropriate, independent action. This will cause the area between the survival curve for disease and disability and that for mortality to compress until, at the extreme, the age at onset of disease and disability is pushed beyond the biologically determined age at death, with the result that people die of senescence free of disease or disability.

One problem with the formulation of the compression of morbidity model presented in the preceding paragraph is that it is hard to define "natural death." Indeed, Fries (1983) has suggested that the dividing line between natural and premature death may be an arbitrary one. Furthermore, the available evidence on the period of terminal decline leading to death suggests that it has not changed as life expectancy at later ages increased, nor is it highly age-variable (e.g., Riley et al., 1985; Roos et al., 1986).

Fries's optimistic argument differs considerably from those of many other investigators. Clearly it is different from the arguments of Feldman (1983) about what we have experienced. Such arguments do not seem to take into account that to achieve the goals set for the adoption of health promotion and disease prevention measures, major efforts are required in some population subgroups, in particular, lower socioeconomic status groups and in some minority groups such as blacks. Nonetheless, it may have utility in defining disability or morbidity prevention goals for selected population groups.

Apart from practical concerns about the pure form of the compression of morbidity model, there are those who propose very different mechanisms for health changes at later ages. For example, Kramer (1981) and Gruenberg (1977) suggest that we are currently increasing the number of years to be spent in morbid and disabled states. This is because they view the bulk of biomedical research as being directed toward reducing mortality and not toward decreasing morbidity and disability. Thus, they suggest that we have effective strategies for moving the mortality curve to the right but not for moving the morbidity and disability curves.

Strehler (1975), in contrast, suggests that we should intervene in the basic aging process. He suggests that within 25 years we should be able to increase the life span by 25 percent. He also suggests that, since we will intervene in basic aging processes, the number of years spent in morbid and disabled states will not increase. Thus, all three curves will move to the right an equal amount so that only the number of person-years spent free of disease (area A) will increase, causing a massive decrease in the ratio of impaired to healthy years.

Each of the above arguments is presented by its respective author as a conceptual model to illustrate a particular perception of the age-changing relation of morbidity, disability, and mortality. For the purposes of actually forecasting likely changes in health status and service needs, we need a more complete and feasible model to accommodate what is being learned from recent epidemiological and biomedical research on aging-related health changes.

The development of the more general model could begin by recognizing that the human organism is subject to multiple pathological processes at later ages. Furthermore, it should be recognized that different diseases have different associated periods of morbidity and disability. For example, cancer has a relatively long morbid period but a short disabled period. Myocardial infarction has short morbid and disabled periods (assuming effective interventions for these diseases exist). Alzheimer's disease has long morbid and disabled periods. Thus, the total morbid and disabled periods for the population can be compressed by targeting interventions to individuals at high risk of the disease processes with the longest disabled periods (assuming effective interventions for these diseases exist). This will change the mix of disease processes operating in the population and may reduce the disabled period more rapidly than life expectancy is increased. This is not to argue that efforts should not continue against the major fatal conditions but instead suggests that inadequate attention has been paid to the potential prevention of the disease processes generating the most disability (e.g., Alzheimer's disease, arthritis, depression). Such a strategy of accelerating compression seems more plausible since it recognizes the multiplicity of chronic conditions affecting the elderly, does not require the concept of natural death, relates interventions to well-defined disease entities, and allows interventions in the disease processes to have effects on life expectancy (i.e., does not require that disease and mortality processes operate independently). It also is arguably a much better representation of our best current scientific evidence. For example, we have little evidence that natural death exists. Autopsy studies of the extreme elderly do report increasing prevalence of multiple chronic diseases at later ages, although it is admittedly more difficult to identify a single cause of death. Nonetheless, interventions in particular disease mechanisms may help to incrementally improve overall system performances.

Verification of results from this type of mortality data also comes from longitudinal studies of aging populations. For example, Lakatta (1985) has studied cardiovascular functioning in the extremely elderly (i.e., persons in their eighties) and found that, in persons free of disease, cardiovascular function could be preserved to advanced ages. Similar evidence has emerged for other organ systems from studies in which individuals with manifest pathological changes have been removed from the analysis. For example, Katzman (1985) discusses the fact that cognitive functions appear to decline very slowly in longitudinally followed populations, especially in persons not close to death. He contrasts these results with those of cross-sectional studies, which show more rapid declines that appear to be artifactual.

Such results are consistent with studies of cause-specific mortality in the United States, which find that the same general mix of diseases is causing mortality at ages that are 2 to 4 years higher on average than they were 15 to 20 years ago. It is also interesting that studies of the variance of the age at death at advanced ages do not show the variance decline with life expectancy increase that would be expected if the upper tail of the age at death distribution were truly being truncated by an absolute biological limit to life span at the current levels of life expectancy.

Although a general model is needed, the model presented in Figure 4.1 is a simplified conceptual framework for studying age changes in the relation of morbidity, disability, and mortality in a population. It has merit because it helps us to understand the changing relation of those health events in a simple framework. Actual analyses will be more complex dealing with the multiplicity of chronic diseases at advanced ages, the possibility of reversals in chronic morbidity and disability, dependent competing risks, the dynamics of human aging processes and risk factors, systematic mortality selection, and the fact that there is a many-to-one mapping between chronic diseases and the type and level of disability.

In addition to analytical issues, the model also raises questions about the nature of data that are required to evaluate the transition. In its simplest form, the model can be evaluated using population life tables, surveys of disability, and epidemiological studies of disease incidence. For example, Wilkins and Adams (1983) used the essence of the concept in assessing active life expectancy gains in the Canadian population. They found that of a 6-year gain in total life expectancy between 1951 and 1978, 4.7 years was in an activity-limited state. Recent life insurance studies suggest that the level of activity limitation was quite low (Blanchet, 1986). More detailed models would involve specific disease processes and their differential contributions to the years lived in each state. Thus, the general concept of the models can help guide us both in terms of needed data and analytic strategies.

DATA NEEDS AND RECOMMENDATIONS

The statistical methodologies and analyses reviewed in this chapter also serve the purpose of identifying critical data needs. In order to describe health transitions at advanced ages, certain specific types of new data are needed and the development of new methodologies for analyzing longitudinal data is required.

One need is for long-term follow-up of well-characterized cohorts. In order to describe health transitions among the elderly it is necessary to have repeated measurements of detailed physiological, social, and health characteristics at advanced ages (i.e., over 75). Such follow-up data would help us to understand the dynamics of physiological aging processes. For example, we might be able to determine whether certain risk factors such as socioeconomic status and overweight cease to be so strongly associated with disease risks at advanced ages, e.g., such follow-up data are necessary to help us disentangle the effects of systematic mortality selection from basic physiological aging processes. A cost-effective approach for generating such measurements at advanced ages would be to make such measurements of existing longitudinal study populations. It is recognized that a full application of the concept advanced may not be feasible, but a limited set of items on physiological and psychosocial functioning could be incorporated in local and national studies. Existing surveys, especially local and national panel studies, can be enhanced by repeated measurement of physiological and psychosocial functioning, capitalizing on the probability sample and baseline measurements available. For example, specific investigation of system functioning, such as cardiovascular function, can benefit by adding studies to existing panel studies with probability samples. Population estimates of physiological parameters at baseline and under conditions of stress (such as a treadmill test) can be derived from such add-on studies to existing cohorts. These data can also be used in longitudinal predictive analyses to enhance usual demographic and self-reported data.

> **Recommendation 4.1:** The panel recommends that detailed physiological assessments be added to existing longitudinal study populations when these cohorts can serve as an appropriate sample to measure specific biological and psychosocial functioning (e.g., cardiovascular status and capacity for daily activities).

Consideration needs to be given to the addition of physiological assessments to the Longitudinal Study on Aging and to community-based special surveys. Examples of community-based epidemiological studies for which follow-up might be done are the Evans County (Cornoni-Huntley et al., 1986) and Alameda County (Berkman and Breslow, 1983) studies. Nationally representative survey populations that might be considered are those in the Longitudinal Retirement History Survey and the National Long-Term Care Study.

A second need is to determine morbidity and mortality risks among nationally representative samples of already morbid and disabled persons. This would help us resolve some of the questions about the effect on society of life expectancy gains at later ages. The prevalence of many chronic diseases is too low to permit the analysis of morbidity and mortality risks for morbid subpopulations using general health surveys. Adequate samples of morbid subpopulations can be obtained by use of a two-stage design in which a large population is screened in the first stage to identify individuals with certain chronic diseases—a target group—followed by a second phase of intensive interviewing of the target group. For example, in 1982 and 1984 a survey was conducted of chronically disabled elderly persons. In that survey persons drawn from the National Health Insurance Master file were screened by telephone to determine if they had a chronic (more than 90 days) ADL or IADL disability. If the answer was yes, then an intensive household survey was done. Screening approximately 36,000 persons identified 6,393 disabled persons. This design provided a cost-effective way to define a disabled subsample that could be followed for future morbidity changes and mortality. Sample members were followed for two years to examine their risk of death, their risk of institutionalization, and the trajectory of change in dependency level. Such data are important in forecasting future health service needs—forecasts that are essential to projecting the costs and resource requirements for health care of the elderly. These projections are required in considering funding and organization of health care.

Recommendation 4.2: The panel recommends that specially focused studies and surveys of specific chronically morbid and disabled elderly populations be conducted.

A third type of useful data could be obtained by systematically extending data collection for clinical studies to measure comorbidities (i.e., multiple morbid conditions). Not only is the issue of comorbidity important for describing normal aging changes, but it is also important for determining what are the appropriate clinical responses to disease at advanced ages. Currently most clinical data bases do not collect extensive data on comorbid conditions. Such data are important for assessing age-related differences in response to different types of medical and surgical treatments.

Recommendation 4.3: The panel recommends that standard guidelines be developed for collecting clinical data on comorbidities at advanced ages and that the National Center for Health Statistics and various institutes of the National Institutes of Health promote the collection of such data in regularly funded clinical study programs.

A fourth requirement is for data that systematically relate chronic disease diagnoses to level and type of disability. This would allow us to generate the mapping functions of diseases to disabilities and to utilize the extensive epidemiological data on disease risk factor associations in forecasting future demand for long-term care services.

Recommendation 4.4: The panel recommends that standard health surveys and epidemiological studies include questions that help clarify the relationship between different diseases and different types and levels of disability at different advanced ages.

Specifically, questions should be included that identify the diseases that are the major causes of different components of functional loss and disability.

A fifth requirement is for increased geographic disaggregation of data. Geographic disaggregation would allow us to take better advantage of naturally occurring population differences in risk. Different subpopulations have very different exposures and disease risks. Such disaggregation would require more detailed tabulation of currently existing data. It is therefore a relatively low-cost way of increasing the usefulness of data that have been collected.

Recommendation 4.5: The panel recommends that more studies and analyses be conducted of the geographic variation of morbidity and mortality risks.

In order to be able to conduct such studies, it will be necessary to examine the question of identifying specific morbidity and mortality events at a level of aggregation detailed enough that the area populations studied are relatively homogeneous. County-level mortality data need to be disaggregated to smaller areas.

Probably no single data source is adequate to study detailed health transitions at advanced ages. The interactions of chronic diseases and aging changes are such complex phenomena that they can best be studied by using information from multiple data sources. This suggests the need for biologically motivated models of the basic physiological processes that can be used to integrate parameter estimates developed from different data sources. Such a strategy for integrating and evaluating multiple data sources must be pursued both as a way of systematizing our knowledge about health dynamics and as a strategy for identifying critical data needs.

Recommendation 4.6:   The panel recommends that the National Institute of Aging and the National Science Foundation conduct or sponsor studies to develop statistical procedures that can utilize multiple data sources for studies of health transitions.

5
Health Promotion and Disease Prevention

INTRODUCTION

Health promotion and disease prevention are a major emerging theme in geriatric medicine and health care generally. Although efforts have typically been targeted at younger persons, there is growing evidence that this approach is both appropriate and feasible for those age 65 and over (Office of Technology Assessment, 1985b). The health promotion and disease prevention approach is one of a number of possible strategies to deal with what has increasingly become a hallmark of current times: the prevalence of chronic illness and multiple chronic illnesses or functional impairments among the elderly. While it will not replace medical care either for the treatment of acute diseases or for acute flare-ups of chronic illness, this approach has promise for reducing the incidence and prevalence of chronic and acute disease among both the general population and the elderly. (See Office of Technology Assessment, Chapters 4 and 5, 1985b; and Kane et al., 1985, for a review of the state of the art in health promotion and disease promotion in the elderly.) In addition, of course, both long-term medical treatment and care for many diseases and illnesses, as well as research to improve diagnosis, treatment, and prevention of chronic and acute disease, are a continuing need.

Selected policy questions relating to health promotion and disease prevention include:

- Should more resources be allocated to increasing our scientific and clinical knowledge base on the efficacy of many health

108

promotion and prevention activities for the elderly population?

- To what extent should public and private programs be developed to motivate older persons who are still asymptomatic to health-maintaining behavior?
- What success rate in modifying health behavior can we anticipate for older patients with various forms of chronic illness or disability?
- What institutions and what professions should be responsible for health promotion? Should health professionals be trained, and should their training be publicly supported?
- How can we move toward a more balanced relationship between the minuscule national investment in health education and other aspects of preventive medicine and the overwhelming resources devoted to medical care directed to reducing the duration and severity of disease and disability?
- Should public and private health insurance programs pay for health promotion and disease prevention interventions?

DEFINITIONS, FEDERAL INITIATIVES, AND GOALS

What is health promotion and disease prevention? Simply stated, health promotion involves "the development of behaviors that improve bodily functioning and enhance an individual's ability to adapt to a changing environment" (Ward, 1984:6). Disease prevention involves actions to reduce or eliminate exposure to risks that might increase the chances that an individual or group will incur disease, disability, or premature death. Some risk factors for disease and disability are mutable or amenable to change (such as personal habits), while others (such as genetic endowment and family history) are not (Kane et al., 1985). A major goal of the health promotion and disease prevention approach—both for individuals and for an entire population—is "to identify the health problems for which preventive efforts can result in more appropriate utilization of health services and improvements in health status" (Lee, 1985:784).

This approach to health emphasizes the importance of lifestyle and personal behavior in improving personal health status and in maintaining health and functioning, both physical and mental. It also recognizes that the extent to which health care interventions and behavior change or channeling can be effective in promoting health and preventing disease depends in part on current health status and the stage in the life cycle in which particular interventions are introduced. Both concepts underscore the need for individuals and family units to accept personal responsibility for their own health and to take the initiative in managing their health care.

Three types of prevention activities can affect health and well-being of the elderly. Primary prevention refers to efforts to eliminate health or functional problems at their source—that is, preventing their occurrence—or to procedures (such as immunizations, improving nutritional status, and increasing physical fitness and emotional well-being) that reduce the incidence of disease or render a population at risk not vulnerable to that risk. Secondary prevention involves efforts to detect adverse health conditions early in their course and to intervene promptly and effectively, or to curtail the spread of disease to others. Tertiary prevention aims to reduce the duration and severity of potentially disabling sequelae of disease and disability, to reduce complications of disease once established, to minimize suffering, and to assist the individual in adjusting to irremediable conditions (see Lowy, 1983; Office of Technology Assessment, 1985b; World Health Organization, 1986; and Chapter 6 of this report).

Federal Initiatives

Interest in health promotion and disease prevention activities nationwide, and in particular for older Americans, has been stimulated by federal initiatives. The first major step was publication of the report by the U.S. Department of Health, Education, and Welfare entitled *Healthy People: The Surgeon General's Report on Health Promotion and Disease Prevention* in 1979. Noting that individual behavior and lifestyle, as well as the environment, are major determinants of health and illness that are amenable to change, the report contends that health promotion and disease prevention are critical to further improvements in health status. The report laid out a set of 5 broad national goals and 15 priority areas for improving the health of the American people during the 1980s. Each goal targeted an age group of the population, from infants to older adults. Health promotion activities initiated before people become elderly would tend to improve their health status in old age. For older adults, the stated goal was "To improve the health and quality of life for older adults and, by 1990, to reduce the average annual number of days of restricted activity due to acute or chronic conditions by 20 percent, to fewer than 30 days per year for people aged 65 and older" (U.S.

Department of Health, Education, and Welfare, 1979). Among the 15 priority areas were high blood pressure control, immunization, surveillance and control of infectious diseases, smoking control, improved nutrition, and physical fitness and exercise. All of these have relevance for the elderly. The perspective for health promotion and disease prevention obviously extends far beyond these goals for 1990.

Subsequent to the publication of the surgeon general's report, the Public Health Service published *Promoting Health/Preventing Disease: Objectives for the Nation* (U.S. Department of Health and Human Services, 1980a), which included separate reports on each of the 15 priority areas. A total of 226 measurable national objectives were presented under 5 major headings: improved health status, reduced risk factors, increased public or professional awareness, improved services or protection, and improved surveillance and evaluation systems. Implementation plans for achieving these objectives were presented in the supplement to the September-October 1983 issue of *Public Health Reports*, entitled *Promoting Health/Preventing Disease: Public Health Service Implementation Plans for Attaining the Objectives for the Nation.* (U.S. Department of Health and Human Services, 1984).

A more recent federal initiative in the area of health promotion and disease prevention is the establishment in 1984 of the U.S. Preventive Services Task Force within the Public Health Service to develop recommendations for the appropriate use of preventive services in clinical settings (see U.S. Department of Health and Human Services, 1984). Another initiative was mandated by the U.S. Congress under P.L. 98-551. This law authorized the Department of Health and Human Services, through its Centers for Disease Control, to establish, maintain, and operate centers for research and demonstration with respect to health promotion and disease prevention (U.S. Congress, 1984). In accordance with this congressional mandate, the Centers for Disease Control in spring 1986 approved the creation of such centers at the Schools of Public Health of the University of North Carolina, the University of Texas, and the University of Washington. In contrast to the other two schools, the University of Washington's center is to focus on the elderly. Although the preceding discussion emphasizes federal initiatives, there are obvious implications for the private sector, for example, in the organization and delivery of services and the financing of medical care.

Goals

Most statements of health promotion and disease prevention goals for the elderly acknowledge that expected outcomes for older persons—especially those who already have chronic illnesses or disabilities—may be different from those for younger persons who do not yet have such illnesses or disabilities. Cure, or full restoration of health or function, may not be a realistic general goal for the elderly. More realistic goals might involve tertiary prevention efforts such as maintenance or stabilization of existing health and function, amelioration of the effects of disease and disability, and postponement or delay of further disability and functional limitation. Even small gains in the ability to maintain current health and to reduce functional disability may make a major difference in the quality of life experienced by an older person. For the elderly population as a whole, shifting or delaying the average age of onset of particular diseases and disabilities, such as hip fracture, may make survival to old age more pleasant, as active life expectancy is increased and morbidity is shifted to the end of the life span. Preservation of personal independence and avoidance of institutionalization may also be viewed as legitimate goals of a health promotion and disease prevention strategy for the elderly, as they are so intimately related to quality of life.

Broadly stated, the goal of health promotion and disease prevention for the elderly may be viewed as the avoidance or delay of "the potentially reversible . . . physical, mental, or social factors that lead to unnecessary functional dependence and institutionalization" (Filner and Williams, 1981).

HEALTH PROMOTION AND DISEASE PREVENTION FOR THE ELDERLY

A note of caution is required before the development of health promotion and disease prevention strategies for the elderly population is enthusiastically endorsed. Attempts to improve the quality of old age require an understanding of the risk factors for common disease among the elderly and the efficacy of strategies to decrease the risk of morbidity. Simplistic generalizations from studies of young and middle age adults to the elderly in this realm are frequently invalid. Middle aged adults and the elderly differ in their patterns of disease and disease presentation.

Furthermore, the elderly represent a select group of survivors, with physiologic alterations that may influence pathophysiologic processes. For instance, the widely cited Alameda County study (Wingard et al., 1982) reported reduced mortality in young and middle-aged adults who never smoked, drank little alcohol, were physically active, and slept seven or eight hours nightly. In contrast, however, in a similar analysis of elderly Massachusetts residents (Branch and Jette, 1984) it was found that five-year mortality rates were not influenced by alcohol intake, physical activity, or sleeping habits, indicating the age modification of risk factors. Similarly, a recent study suggests that more overweight elderly subjects have a lower rather than a higher mortality rate from coronary disease (Jajich et al., 1984). This controversial finding is difficult to explain in view of the known adverse effects of obesity on diabetes, hypertension, and hyperlipidemia and indicates a need for detailed evaluation of the potential protective effect of moderate overweight in old age (the two preceding paragraphs closely parallel Rowe, 1985:828).

There are several reasons for adopting a health promotion and disease prevention approach for the elderly, despite legitimate cautions. Among them are the plasticity of the aging process; the possibility of modifying physiologic or pathologic conditions that, although associated with so-called normal aging, also entail risks to health; and the high incidence of chronic disease among the elderly, which increases the importance of postponing additional disability. Furthermore, life expectancy is increasing and it is desirable to enhance health status during these additional years of life.

The Plasticity of the Aging Process

The health effects of deleterious habits and lifestyles are typically cumulative, and for this reason often viewed as nonremediable—making primary prevention among younger members of the population appear as a preferable strategy for improving the nation's health. There is, however, increasing evidence to suggest that some harmful habits and behaviors are capable of modification and even reversal, sometimes when interventions and changes occur late in life. Recent studies on osteoporosis, for example, indicate that moderate exercise can retard age-related bone loss and even in some cases increase bone density in elderly women, including women in their nineties and those living in institutions (Aloia et al., 1978; Smith and Reddan, 1976; Smith et al., 1981).

Risks Associated With Normal Aging

There is evidence to suggest that physiologic or pathologic changes so common with advancing age as to be considered normal by clinicians may not be without risk. Although systolic blood pressure increases with age among the American elderly population, it is also clear that increases in systolic blood pressure are associated with marked increases in the risk of stroke and coronary heart disease (Rowe, 1983). Just because a finding is considered normal among the elderly does not mean that it is also harmless. Perhaps the term *usual aging* should be substituted for *normative aging*, to recognize the possibility of adverse effects associated with typical age-related change and the importance of considering techniques to modify these usual, but not necessarily harmless, characteristics.

The High Incidence of Chronic Disease and Illness Among the Elderly

While persons of any age may have chronic disease or disability (e.g., both children and adults become deaf or blind, acquire permanent orthopedic disabilities and develop degenerative diseases requiring continuing treatment and care), the elderly are particularly vulnerable to chronic disease and disability. An estimated 86 percent of persons over age 65 have one or more chronic diseases (Office of Technology Assessment, 1985b). Among the noninstitutionalized elderly, who have a much lower prevalence of severe limitations and dependency than the institutionalized elderly, some 46 percent had arthritis, 37 percent had hypertension, 28 percent had a hearing loss, and 28 percent had a heart condition in 1981 (Office of Technology Assessment, 1985b; Rice, 1986). Therefore, efforts to maintain existing health and well-being, to ameliorate the effects of illness and disability, and to delay or postpone further disability are particularly important for the elderly population.

Increases in Average Life Expectancy and Individual Variability

The life expectancy of the elderly is increasing. Those currently age 65 can expect on average to live another 16 years (more than 14 for men and 18 for women) (Office of Technology Assessment, 1985b:10). With increasing longevity, current elderly cohorts, as well as younger age groups, can be expected to live through longer periods of exposure to risk factors, including those posed by the environment, diet and nutrition, and personal behavior and lifestyle, and will have more time to develop symptoms than past generations. Furthermore, as with other age groups, there is great variability in the health and functional status of older persons. While some are severely debilitated or ill and can benefit minimally if at all from preventive interventions, others are thriving and show no evidence of disease or disability.

CRITICAL ISSUES

Five issues are of current concern in the health promotion and disease prevention approach to health care: (1) the inconclusiveness of the scientific and clinical evidence of the efficacy of many promotion and prevention activities, (2) the need for additional knowledge concerning factors that facilitate behavior modification among persons of all ages, (3) the shortage of health care personnel trained in this approach, (4) the potential impact that accelerating growth in the number and utilization of health maintenance organizations and other systems with prepaid capitation fees will have on this approach to health care, and (5) the effect that prospective payment systems, as exemplified by diagnosis-related groups for the elderly under Medicare, will have on the services received.

The scientific basis for many of the health promotion and disease prevention activities currently in vogue is inadequate. With respect to the elderly in particular, there is only modest evidence that particular behaviors and interventions can prevent disease or retard the impact of illness and disability, once established. For example, the role of exercise in reducing the risk of coronary heart disease and stroke for women and the elderly is not yet known (Office of Technology Assessment, 1985b). Similarly, it is not yet understood whether current obesity or a history of chronic obesity is a risk factor for coronary heart disease (Office of Technology Assessment, 1985b). And the relative risks and benefits of different levels of exercise for older persons—particularly those with chronic disease—have not yet been established (Office of Technology Assessment, 1985b). Nonetheless, a variety of activities and behavior changes have been widely advertised as health promoting and disease preventing—as ways to avoid everything from cancer to heart disease. Private-sector initiatives in the area of physical fitness, nutrition, and diet counseling have been largely responsible here, although the scientific and clinical evidence on which much of the popularized advice to the public and to individuals is based is often inconclusive or conflicting.

A related issue is the need for increased knowledge of the factors that facilitate attitude and behavior change among the population as a whole and among segments of it, including the elderly (Franks et al., 1983; Sanazaro, 1985). An effective national strategy of prevention and promotion, such as that established by the Public Health Service initially with the publication of *Healthy People: The Surgeon General's Report on Health Promotion and Disease Prevention* (U.S. Department of Health, Education, and Welfare, 1979), depends not only on knowledge of scientific and clinical efficacy of particular interventions but also on the ability and willingness of individuals to modify their behavior.

A third issue is the shortage of physicians and other health personnel who are trained to provide health promotion and disease prevention services to their patients (Lee, 1985). One reason for this shortage is the passive structure of the U.S. health care delivery system, which generally relies on individuals to present themselves to physicians and other providers when and if they have a problem. Until very recently, health care coverage for most people, and Medicare reimbursement policies for the elderly, have reinforced a system of health care that creates no demand for health promotion and disease prevention practitioners. Medicare has not generally covered individuals or compensated providers of care for prevention and promotion activities.

Two developments that may affect the rate at which the health promotion and disease prevention approach gains widespread acceptance are the recent dramatic growth in the number and utilization of prepaid health plans by the general public and by the elderly and the provision of coverage and reimbursement for Medicare enrollees and providers of care involved in health plans that are paid prospectively according to a fixed rate capitation formula. HMOs, one type of capitated plan, provide a comprehensive range of medical or health care services within a single organization in exchange for a fixed monthly or annual fee. As their name suggests, HMOs might be expected to encourage their enrollees to maintain health and prevent disease through the particular variety of services they offer and the gatekeeping functions they perform to reduce utilization of more expensive forms of care (such as hospitalization). Information on the extent to which these functions are carried out would be important. From June

1983 to June 1985, enrollment in HMOs increased by 20 percent per year, with an estimated 8 percent of the U.S. population—or some 19 million persons—enrolled as of June 1985 (Tarlov, 1986:29-30). In 1985 the Health Care Financing Administration issued regulations that encourage HMOs to enroll Medicare beneficiaries on a capitation basis (Ginsburg and Hackbarth, 1986).

DATA NEEDS

This portion of the chapter discusses existing federal surveys that provide data relevant to health promotion and disease prevention for the general population and for the elderly. These surveys are reviewed from two perspectives: the extent to which they provide information about the health promotion and disease prevention knowledge and activities of the general population (including the elderly), and the extent to which they provide information about the health promotion and disease prevention activities of providers of care (such as physicians and nurses). Population-based surveys yield information by surveying samples of individuals selected from the general population or certain segments of it, such as minorities, the elderly, or women of childbearing age. Provider-based surveys survey individual or institutional providers of care, such as physicians or nursing homes.

Public Knowledge About Health Promotion and Disease Prevention

The success of a health promotion or health maintenance and disease prevention program depends on many things. One is an informed and knowledgeable public, which in turn depends on widespread dissemination of the known benefits and harmful effects to health and well-being of particular behaviors. Also necessary is a willingness on the part of individuals to change attitudes, habits, and behaviors—often long-standing ones—and the initiative to undertake responsibility for one's own health and the health of one's family.

More information is needed about the techniques and strategies that are likely to be effective in inducing and maintaining attitude and behavior change, not only among the elderly, but also among the general population. In fact, there is a considerable amount of research in the area of behavior modification techniques under way at present and planned for the future—some of it experimental, involving controlled clinical trials, and some of it less rigorous in nature (see, for example, Russell, 1987).

There is also concrete evidence demonstrating that successful campaigns to educate the public, increase its awareness of the harmful effects of particular practices, and motivate individuals to take action can be mounted. A prominent example is the successful National High Blood Pressure Education Program launched by the National Heart Institute in 1972 to spread the word to physicians, their patients, and to ordinary citizens (U.S. Department of Health and Human Services, 1985).

In 1985, the National Health Interview Survey (National Center for Health Statistics, 1985a) described in Chapter 3 included a health promotion and disease prevention supplement as an effort to obtain information on the knowledge and behaviors of the general public. The supplement included questions pertinent to various age groups including the elderly. For example, adult respondents were asked about their knowledge of factors that increase one's chances of developing heart disease and stroke, about foods associated with high blood pressure, about diseases caused by smoking and alcohol, and about activities that prevent tooth decay and gum disease, among others (National Center for Health Statistics, 1985a). The supplement thus provides data relevant to the Public Health Service's goals and objectives for promoting health and preventing disease (U.S. Department of Health and Human Services, 1980a) and the implementation plans for attaining the objectives for the nation (U.S. Department of Health and Human Services, 1983).

Despite the obvious importance of health maintenance and disease prevention, data are not routinely available through national data systems on the extent to which the population is informed as to the causes of preventable illnesses and conditions and the actions they might take to reduce their own risks of developing such illnesses and accompanying impairments.

As noted earlier, the health needs and concerns of the elderly are somewhat different from those of younger persons, because of their stage in the life cycle, their social circumstances, and the fact that the risk of particular diseases and disabilities changes with age and with the existing health and functional status of the individual. Separate health promotion and disease prevention modules (clusters of items on specific topics) should be developed that are appropriate to the elderly and subgroups of this population, since risk factors and expected health and functional outcomes for particular diseases and disabilities among the elderly vary. Modules should be designed to reflect special conditions among racial and ethnic minorities, the poor, residents of rural areas, women, the oldest-old, the impaired and institutionalized, and those elderly who are at high risk for or who have particular diseases or disabilities. The panel also believes that such modules and items that have a more narrow focus on a particular disease or disability for which the elderly are at greater risk than the rest of the population should also be developed, to be administered in or along with selected population surveys. It would be useful to develop modules and information items for subjects such as breast self-examination and screening, pap tests, and osteoporosis prevention and retardation for women; issues of falling (including items on hip fracture and broken bones); primary prevention activities such as influenza and tetanus shots for the institutionalized and other immunizations and their purposes; incontinence; adverse effects of drugs; social isolation, depression, and other potentially preventable and/or remediable social and emotional conditions; the role of diet, nutrition, and exercise in the prevention or retardation of particular illnesses; and the use of preventive safety measures in the home.

Both the National Health Interview Survey and the National Health and Nutrition Examination Surveys would be good vehicles for health promotion and disease prevention items and modules for the general population and for the elderly. Both surveys are described in Chapter 3 of this report. The NHANES, scheduled to be fielded again in 1988 (NHANES III) is a unique opportunity because of its inclusion of physiologic measures in addition to self-reported (interview) information on health and nutrition status and practices.

A major policy issue is whether the federal government should fund health promotion and disease prevention activities and, if so, which ones. To clarify this issue, information is needed on the extent to which population subgroups of the elderly are informed about health promotion and disease prevention practices and the degree to which persons of all ages behave in ways known to promote health and prevent illness. Such information is also needed to assess changes in the extent of such activities resulting from public and private initiatives.

Recommendation 5.1: The panel recommends (a) that modules of health promotion and disease prevention items (including those concerned with attitudes, knowledge, and behavior) be developed that are appropriate for the elderly and subgroups of the elderly population that are at risk for particular diseases, illnesses, disabilities, or conditions, which can be used with a variety of population-based surveys; (b) that these health promotion and disease prevention survey modules be tested on relevant segments of the elderly population; and (c) that successful modules be incorporated in population-based surveys such as the National Health Interview Survey and the National Health and Nutrition Examination Survey, or as supplements to them.

Development of these modules will require cooperation and coordination of effort by several agencies, including the Office of Health Promotion and Disease Prevention, the National Center for Health Services Research and Health Care Technology, the National Center for Health Statistics, and institutes within the National Institutes of Health.

The Role of Physicians

Once the scientific basis for particular health promotion and disease prevention interventions and behaviors has been established, and the medical and health care technology to implement them has been developed, physicians and other health care personnel can play important roles in promoting health and preventing disease, with patients of all ages, including the elderly.

The elderly, on average, make more visits to physicians annually than middle-aged persons. In 1985, for example, persons ages 65-74 averaged 7.7 physician visits per year, and those age 75 and over had an average of 9.3 visits per year, in contrast with 6.1 visits per year for persons ages 45-64 (National Center for Health Statistics, 1986b). In 1979 elders (age 65 and older) with chronic activity limitation averaged 8.7 physician visits per year, in contrast with 4.3 visits per year for those without activity limitation. Only 5 percent of the elderly had not seen a physician for five or more years (Rice, 1986). The sheer frequency with which the typical older person visits a physician, particularly since the elderly tend to see the same physician (Rice, 1986), enhances the possibility of physician influence.

Although some patients, including elderly patients, do not adhere to physician-prescribed regimens such as drug regimens, it has been shown that in the area of promoting and maintaining attitude and behavior change, physicians—particularly primary care physicians—can be effective (German et al., 1982; U.S. Department of Health and Human Services, 1986c; Gilson et al., 1984). This is especially true when other intervention techniques, such as providing the patient with written material on the issue in question, are used in conjunction with physician-initiated discussion. This was demonstrated in a recent study conducted at a large Seattle-area health maintenance organization in which researchers examined the relative impact of strategies involving physician-patient discussions and other intervention methods on compliance with colorectal screening and smoking cessation (Gilson et al., 1984). For colorectal screening compliance, the most effective intervention was a three-step strategy consisting of a physician-patient talk about the importance of the screening test, sending a postcard as a reminder, and calling those who failed to return the test within 10 days. With respect to smoking cessation, experimental interventions involving physician discussions with patients, together with the provision of self-help material, achieved a higher rate of compliance with trying to quit smoking than did other interventions. None of the interventions, however, were notably successful in achieving smoking cessation (Gilson et al., 1984).

A major drawback to fully exploiting the potential influence of physicians in health promotion and disease prevention among their patients has been the paucity of data on the extent to which physicians currently do engage in prevention activities. Such activities might include screening examinations and inoculations, discussion and counseling, and therapeutic measures and follow-up where efficacy measures have been scientifically and clinically established.

The mechanism being used to determine some aspects of physician behavior in this area is the National Ambulatory Medical Care Survey (also discussed in Chapter 9). This survey, conducted annually from 1973 through 1981, and again in 1985, with three-year periodicity planned for the future, collects data on office visits made by ambulatory patients to nonfederal physicians who are principally employed in office-based patient care practice. The nature of the physician-patient encounter is recorded for a sample of patient visits to a sample of such physicians in the coterminous United States. The physician sample is drawn from files maintained by the American Medical Association and the American Osteopathic Association. In 1985, the latest year for which data are available, some 3,500 physicians (70.2 percent of those sampled) participated in the survey. Of the 71,594 physician-patient visits sampled and recorded, 14,700 (20.5 percent) were by people age 65 and over (National Center for Health Statistics, 1987b).

At present, the data collected on the physician-patient encounter include the date and duration of the visit, the reason(s) for the visit (the patient's presenting complaints or symptoms), the physician's diagnoses, whether the major problem is new or previously addressed by this physician, the diagnostic and therapeutic services ordered or provided, and the action at the end of the visit. The patient record for this survey provides a checklist for the physician that distinguishes between medication and nonmedication therapy (including among other things psychotherapy, diet counseling, and other counseling). The 1985 patient record report of the visit also contains checkoff items on specific tests, e.g., blood pressure, glucose tolerance, visual acuity, and breast examination. These sections need to be reexamined to increase their usefulness in identifying specific health promotion and disease prevention activities. At present, such activities cannot be distinguished from those carried out as a follow-up for previously diagnosed disease or because of suspected disease.

The panel recognizes the space constraints of the form currently being used for the National Ambulatory Medical Care Survey, but we believe that changes can be accommodated in the items currently included and a distinction made between prevention and treatment. The recommendation below recognizes that:

- physicians and other health care providers play a critical role in influencing the behavior of their patients,
- the health needs of the elderly often differ from those of the remainder of the population, and
- some diseases and illnesses of old age can be modified through prevention and health promotion.

Recommendation 5.2:   The panel recommends that the National Center for Health Statistics: (a) develop questions pertaining to the health promotion and disease prevention practices of health care providers that include categories with special relevance for the elderly to be used in provider-based surveys and that (b) these questions be included in the National Ambulatory Medical Care Survey to obtain information on physician-patient encounters.

These questions should ascertain: (1) the activities that physicians undertake to change patients' behavior and increase their awareness and understanding of health promotion and disease prevention, (2) the specific preventive measures (such as dietary advice and screening for hypertension) taken during the patient visit, and (3) information obtained on changes in patient's behavior.

A recommendation in Chapter 9 to expand the sampling frame of the National Ambulatory Medical Care Survey to include additional physician types and practice settings is pertinent here as well.

Providers of Health Maintenance and Disease Prevention Services to the Elderly

Many different kinds of physicians, for example, family practitioners, pediatricians, internists, psychiatrists, and cardiologists, engage in some kinds of health promotion and disease prevention activities with their patients, but the extent to which they do so varies and is currently unknown. A recent report on the 1980-1981 National Ambulatory Medical Care Survey (National Center for Health Statistics, 1984b) points out some differences by type of physician and age and condition of patient, for instance, in the extent to which a blood pressure reading is taken during an office visit and whether medication or nonmedication therapy (e.g., counseling) is provided. However, this survey, as currently constituted, does not attempt to fully document physician practices in health promotion or maintenance and disease prevention. Nor is this survey designed to ascertain the extent to which different physician specialties and other providers of care consider health promotion and disease prevention concerns as among the services they should provide to their patients.

Many other types of practitioners, such as nutritionists and social workers, also provide health and health-related services to persons of all ages, including the elderly. Furthermore, health promotion and disease prevention services are also provided in a variety of nonmedical settings, including physical fitness centers and senior centers by professional, paraprofessional, and nonprofessional support personnel.

Comprehensive information on the numbers of professionals and allied health personnel who provide health promotion and disease prevention services to the elderly in a variety of settings does not exist. While some federal agencies such as the Bureau of Health Professions of the Health Resources and Services Administration (U.S. Public Health Service) collect data on health manpower and/or health manpower training (see, for instance, Fifth Report to the President and Congress: U.S. Department of Health and Human Services, 1986a), none of them collects information on professionals and allied personnel who render health promotion and disease prevention services to the U.S. population at large or to the elderly. Although some data exist on members of health maintenance organizations and their enrollment figures (which are in flux because of rapid growth in this area), there are no comprehensive data on the services HMOs provide and the numbers of elderly who receive these services as HMO enrollees.

The Health Research Extension Act of 1985, Section 8, called for a study of personnel for health needs of the elderly. It directed the secretary of the U.S. Department of Health and Human Services to "conduct a study on the adequacy and availability of personnel to meet the current and projected health needs (including needs for home and community-based care) of elderly Americans through the year 2020." The National Institute on Aging, in a joint effort with the Health Resources and Services Administration, conducted the study, with its director acting as chair of a committee that includes representatives from several federal agencies (see National Institute on Aging, 1985, and Chapter 9 of this report for more information). The secretary's report, submitted to Congress in fall 1987, includes recommendations related to the number of primary care physicians, dentists, and other health personnel needed to provide adequate care for the elderly; the education and training needs of other physicians, dentists, and health personnel to provide care responsive to the particular needs of the elderly, and the financing of geriatric and training activities (U.S. Department of Health and Human Services, 1987). While the study addresses the manpower and training needs for many different types of health personnel who provide care to the elderly, it does not focus explicitly on the area of health promotion and disease prevention, although it recognizes it as a special issue area. The Office of Disease Prevention and Health Promotion within the Department's Public Health Service also does not routinely collect data on the numbers of health personnel involved in health promotion and disease prevention services to the elderly or on their training in this area. The panel believes such information is important to determine whether there is need for additional trained personnel and training programs for health promotion and disease prevention among the elderly.

Recommendation 5.3: The panel recommends that the Bureau of Health Professions collect information on health care personnel (including professionals and support staff such as nurse's aides) who focus on health promotion and disease prevention activities and services to the elderly in a variety of medical and nonmedical, and institutional and noninstitutional, settings. Estimates of the numbers of such personnel and their health promotion and disease prevention activities should be ascertained.

6

Quality of Care

National data systems have been a largely underdeveloped source of information for measuring quality of care among the elderly. There are compelling reasons for identifying needs for this type of information and the extent to which such systems could meet them. The Office of Technology Assessment (1985a:77) points out that "Medicare's prospective payment system (PPS) has intensified concern with the complex relationship between cost and quality of medical care" and that "assessing PPS impacts on quality of care is critical." Among the reasons given is that, if PPS succeeds as a cost containment strategy, "its effect on the quality of care will be a deciding factor in the program's continual survival." Another report (Institute of Medicine, 1986) focuses on the importance of information systems for assessing and improving the quality of care of nursing home residents and recommends (p. 43) that the secretary of the Department of Health and Human Services "undertake a study to design a system of acquiring and using resident assessment data."

These reports reflect the emergence of quality of care as a matter of central interest for policies directed at controlling costs or improving services for specific subgroups of the elderly. The larger context consists of an agenda of policies concerned with the application of prospective payment systems to sectors other than hospital care, modifications in Medicare and Medicaid benefits, and availability of staff, facilities, and alternative sources of care, particularly for the long-term care patient.

Policies that have been adopted, or are being contemplated, may have both short-term and long-term effects on quality of care, but the character of these effects is not clear. The potential for differential effects exists because of the diversity of health care systems; the increasing competition among providers; and the heterogeneity of the elderly population. The elderly vary in their health and mental health care needs, social and economic status, and living arrangements—circumstances subject to rapid change as age advances (Shanas and Maddox, 1985). The utility of information on quality of care for national policy purposes is directly related to the ability to examine relationships involving these variables.

Selected policy questions relating to the quality of care, listed in order from issues that require research or evaluations to questions that depend on or are related to measurement of quality of care, include:

- Should quality assurance mechanisms for health care services of the elderly be strengthened because of the adverse effects of cost containment?
- Should Professional Review Organizations (PROs) under Medicare be strengthened to ensure quality of care for Medicare beneficiaries?
- To what extent should government and private insurance programs regulate quality of care under their reimbursement mechanisms?
- How has the change in Medicare's payment system to DRGs affected the quality of care for elderly patients?
- Has the emergence of competitive health maintenance organizations (HMOs) provided economic incentives for their elderly enrollees or affected the quality of care provided to them? Who should be responsible for monitoring quality of care in HMOs?
- How can we develop, refine, and implement improved and standardized measurements of quality of care for older people? Who should be responsible?

The discussion that follows presents the framework within which quality of care is most often examined, identifies several measures of quality of care suitable for national data systems, and considers steps needed to ensure availability of such measures.

A FRAMEWORK FOR QUALITY OF CARE ASSESSMENT

It is now possible to talk about a generation of effort to progress from broad definitions of quality of care to the identification of criteria that can be applied to measure quality. Although specific details of quality of care assessment have varied, the framework that is most widely accepted consists of three components—structure, process, and outcome (Donabedian, 1980). Primary emphasis in explicating these concepts has been directed at the diagnosis and management of illness and is focused on transactions between providers and patients to achieve an appropriate balance of health benefits and risks.

This is clearly an essential aspect of quality of care and is exemplified by approaches taken by Professional Review Organizations in developing programs for quality assurance of inpatient care for Medicare beneficiaries (Mohr, 1985). Other aspects of quality of care that require greater prominence and that are readily accommodated within the categories, structure, process, and outcome, are oriented toward prevention and a consideration of how a system of care is functioning, not only with respect to those who appear for care at the time they do so, but also in terms of the need that exists in a community or general population. Quality is affected by both the technical performance of providers and the extent to which a system reaches those in need, for example, hypertensives under treatment may have high levels of control, but on a population basis there may be a high prevalence of uncontrolled hypertension.

The usual formulation of what is included under each category is given below, expanded to cover some of these considerations.

Structure refers to relatively stable parts of the health care system, such as numbers, types, and qualifications of professional personnel, physical facilities, and medical technologies; it also includes organization and distribution of different types of services, proximity to the population being served, and other factors affecting access to care.

Process refers to what is done to and for the patient or a defined population and how it is done; this includes the application of preventive, diagnostic, and therapeutic procedures, nursing and home care, counseling, referral practices, and coordination of care, follow-up, and monitoring procedures.

Outcome refers to changes in health status or maintenance of desirable levels of health influenced by health services; this includes one or more dimensions of physical and psychosocial functioning, disability, prevention of disease or complication of disease, satisfaction with health care, and mortality.

A comprehensive assessment of quality of care would be concerned with all three components and their interrelationship, with the ultimate measure of quality determined by the outcome of care (Kessner et al., 1973). In practice, there are often severe constraints in linking particular structural factors and processes of care to specific measures of health status. Standards for many elements of structure are based on professional judgments and are used for such purposes as accreditation, licensing, Medicare certifications, and establishing qualifications for staff in, for example, hospitals, group practices, and nursing homes. However, standards do not always represent a consensus; they are subject to change as new knowledge is acquired and new technology developed, and different structural patterns may achieve similar levels of quality. Furthermore, the fact that standards are met does not provide assurance that a favorable effect on health status will follow. In short, structural factors such as the availability of highly qualified primary care providers, specialists and support services, or regionalized emergency medical service systems may increase the probability of receiving high-quality care, but they are not sufficient conditions for determining quality.

Process of care measures provide more generally accepted indicators of quality of care, reflecting as they do what care is delivered and how. The measures are derived mainly from professional norms of practice or research in which some link to outcome is implicitly or explicitly expected, whether this is improved functioning, delay in dependency, or relief from pain or depression. The degree of certainty about a link may be weak in some cases because of lack of information about the natural history of disease, the relative effectiveness of alternative treatment modalities, or the role of behavioral and biological characteristics of patients in determining the course of illness. The selection of process measures for assessing quality of care seeks to minimize these limitations. Measures are available or being developed that range from adherence to algorithms for the treatment of specific conditions (Greenfield et al., 1981) to communication and counseling (Inui and Carter, 1985), detection of need for health services (Aday and Andersen, 1975; Shapiro et al., 1985), matching need with appropriate sources of care in acute episodes of illness and in long-term care, for which coordination of services is important (Mathematica Policy Research, Inc., 1986).

The pessimism that long pervaded the outlook for having outcome measures to assess quality of care has been replaced by a more optimistic view. Although there are many uncertainties about how health status is influenced by personal and social factors, knowledge has cumulated regarding the effectiveness of specific health care interventions. Advances have been made in the development, testing, and application of health status measures to supplement indices of mortality that are useful in examining both technical and health care system effects on the health of a population (Bergner, 1985; Brook and Lohr, 1985). This holds true for all age groups, but it is particularly relevant for the elderly, whose needs for health services are high and large proportions of whom could be affected positively or negatively.

We specify outcome measures under the three functional goals of health care below:

Caring involves reassurance and relief from anxiety, satisfaction, and communication between provider and patient, which may affect whether regimens prescribed are followed and response to symptoms and care-seeking are appropriate.

Curing and maintenance involve a reduction in symptoms and dependency, avoidance of complications and iatrogenic effects of treatment and reversing the effects when they occur, improvement or stabilization in functional capacity, and reduction in avoidable mortality. Many specific conditions are candidates for observation, such as hypertension, angina, hip fractures, major depression, glaucoma, cataracts, respiratory diseases, and hearing, visual, and dental defects.

Functional status measures detailed in Chapter 3 represent a spectrum of physical, emotional, and social indicators of health status. They reflect the results of an interaction between population and environmental conditions and processes of care determined by how the delivering system and individual practitioners function. This type of interaction affects aspects of health care such as matching need with demand as affected by availability and access to care, timeliness of medical intervention, planning of long-term care and post-hospital care, coordination of multiple sources of care, and continuity of care.

Prevention measures are designed to prevent, delay, or reverse the progression of disease, and reduce functional limitation, handicap, or dependency due to health conditions. A preventive measure may be interpreted as a surrogate or intermediate outcome measure when its effect on a health condition or health status has been established, when it reaches the population that is at risk and can benefit from it, and when there is appropriate follow-up.

The potential and limitations of what can be gained from specific measures are discussed in Chapter 5. A full treatment of prevention would consider degrees of certainty about efficacy, cost-effectiveness of particular prevention measures, state of readiness among providers to apply them, and method and frequency of the interventions. However, the application of prevention procedures that are generally viewed as desirable would serve as an indicator of quality of care. These include examination and follow-up of asymptomatic individuals for such conditions as hypertension, visual defects, impaired hearing, hypercholesteremia and counseling on smoking cessation, exercise, rest, diet, and rehabilitation aimed at restoring function consistent with the maximum achievable level.

THE ROLE OF NATIONAL INFORMATION SYSTEMS

National data systems have the capacity to produce information needed to derive quality of care measures to determine how quality varies within the population and how it may be influenced by sources of care and policies that affect services received. Many of the specific items required are included in surveys that are already operational or about to start; others are dependent on the extension of existing items or the introduction of new ones.

Additional efforts will be needed to develop and test new measures of outcome and processes of care, as well as methods for making reliable and valid observations on the elderly who are well and those who are infirm or cognitively impaired. In this regard, particular attention needs to be given to methodology and research pertaining to cognitive aspects of survey design, i.e., aspects of survey research interviews pertaining to cognitive processes such as understanding language, remembering and forgetting, perception, judgment, and inferring causes. One direction for such activity is the specification of better questions as well as better ways of expressing questions with respect to cognitive considerations (Fienberg et al., 1985; Lessler and Sirken, 1985). Another is the use of flagging procedures by interviewers to indicate their degree of belief in the correctness of reported responses. Such information could then play a helpful role in the evaluation of the sensitivity of estimates to possibly varying levels of data accuracy. Methodology for expressing the results of such efforts in terms of bias or accuracy also needs better development.

A significant expansion in the measurement of quality of care can be achieved before results of new research are available through the use of currently available or readily adaptable measures, linkage of multiple data sets, and longitudinal information systems. Implementation of the recommendations in earlier sections of this report on health status and health promotion, as well as those in later sections on utilization and long-term care, would achieve this purpose. The additional requirement is a coherent strategy for placing the measures in a quality of care framework.

In developing this strategy, it is important to bear in mind that national information systems should have the capacity to measure quality directly. They should also provide broad indicators of quality of care that can signal that other sources of information are needed (Rutstein et al., 1976). For example, an alert was signaled in 1986 when the Health Care Financing Administration (HCFA) released hospital mortality rates derived from the Medicare hospital bills. The result was to focus attention on how patients are managed in the hospital. Another effect should be to intensify the development of severity of illness measures that are feasible for inclusion in data systems on hospital discharges (Horn and Horn, 1986).

Indicators of quality of care would become more readily available with the adoption of the Long-Term Health Care Minimum Data Set (U.S. Department of Health and Human Services, 1980b), and this would provide a basis for probing more fully into processes of care in institutional and noninstitutional settings. Also relevant for the development of quality of care measures are the recommendations of the Institute of Medicine's Committee on Improving Nursing Home Care for a study to determine the scope and design of an information system useful for regulating nursing homes effectively and considering policies for long-term care (Institute of Medicine, 1986). Quality of care represents a major interest; the results will also be valuable for other data systems.

A concerted effort is needed to develop quality of care measures on the elderly suitable for national information systems. A task force should be established to serve as the locus for this effort. The task force could be the responsibility of the National Committee on Vital and Health Statistics, the Health Information Policy Council in the Department of Health and Human Services, or the Forum on Aging-Related Statistics, the coordinating council of principal government agencies concerned with the provision and use of information on aging. Special expertise and experience will be required, and the task force activity will need to be paralleled by funding of methodological studies through research grants and contracts. The task force should be concerned with assessments of structure, process, and outcome of care for subgroups of the population, with a special emphasis on outcomes of care influenced by delivery system and provider characteristics. Consideration should be given to measures and methods that have the capability of identifying rapidly possible effects of health policy decisions.

Items contained in several of the national health surveys can be used as building blocks for developing quality of care measures. Candidates are found in the NHIS and its supplement on aging and prevention, the NNHS, the NHANES, and the NAMCS, all of which are NCHS surveys; in the Long-Term Care Survey (HCFA and the Office of the Assistant Secretary for Health, DHHS), and in the forthcoming NMES (NCHSR and HCFA). These items should be reexamined for modification, amplification, and replacement based on results of analysis.

> **Recommendation 6.1:** The panel recommends that agencies having cognizance of national data systems, whether based on administrative records or survey data: (1) jointly review these data systems to identify items that can be used in developing quality of care measures and identify missing items that are needed to produce such measures and (2) make provision for collecting the data needed to fill gaps and for producing quality of care measures.

Priority should also be given to development of new items on functional status (as recommended in Chapter 3) and their adoption once they have been tested. The Long-Term Health Care Minimum Data Set (discussed in Chapter 7), should be incorporated into relevant data systems. Appendix D lists the items contained in this minimum data set.

Indicators of quality of care can also be developed by linking data obtained in surveys to other files, such as the National Death Index, or by reinterviews to obtain information on a completed episode of illness.

> **Recommendation 6.2:** The panel recommends that multiple data sources be linked to provide indicators of quality of care during episodes of illness and that continuous, longitudinal data be developed to track the flow of individuals through episodes of illness to recovery, dependency, or death, including their patterns of use of acute and long-term care facilities and community and home care services.

Continued support should be ensured for steps already taken, such as the conduct of the National Mortality Followback Survey; provision for searches of the National Death Index over long periods for deaths among people identified in sample surveys of the NCHS; and follow-up of individuals in the NHANES, the NHIS, and the Long-Term Care Survey; HCFA's Medicare Automatic Data Retrieval System should be completed and continued annually; quality of care assessments of hospital prospective payment systems need to be concerned with pre- and post-hospital care; and urgent attention should be given to the introduction of severity of illness measures.

The panel recognizes that most elderly are capable of responding for themselves when interviewed, but it is uncertain whether issues affecting the quality of information provided by them are similar or different from those at younger age groups. Interviewers encounter additional data quality problems in surveying the elderly because, with advancing age and for many in nursing homes, the number of cognitively impaired people increases and the interviewer is dependent on proxy respondents. The validity of data from proxies may be affected by many factors not well understood at this time. Research on these issues will need to address not only the magnitude and characteristics of the problems involved, but also the methods and sources for improving the quality of the data.

Recommendation 6.3: The panel recommends that the National Center for Health Statistics develop methods for increasing the validity and reliability of health data (health status, needs, and care received) collected in surveys of the elderly, whether from elderly respondents themselves, from their caregivers or next-of-kin, or from both.

7
Long-term Care

INTRODUCTION

People with long-term health problems are a large and increasing proportion of the population of the United States. The elderly are not the only users and potential clients of long-term care. Such people are of all ages and include not only the chronically ill and the infirm but also the physically impaired, the mentally ill, and the mentally retarded. The long-term client tends to use multiple services, both formal and informal, at a time when his or her coping abilities may be increasingly limited because of functional impairment and disability (Murnaghan, 1976). The client may or may not have family and friends to help with caretaking. Among the elderly there is often no one to fill this role.

The needs of the client range from those that are solely medical to those that are basically social. Limited efforts are being made to combine the resources of the medical care and social service systems in support of the long-term care client. At the same time, there is rising concern about the financial burden of long-term care. The number and complexity of client needs and the variety of institutions and agencies through which services are delivered create problems for the client, the caretaker (if there is one), and for policy makers who make decisions about the provision, use, and financing of long-term care. This chapter concentrates on data essential to policy decision making in the area of long-term care of the elderly. Selected policy questions include:

- What is the appropriate mix of services to enable long-term clients to be maintained at their maximum levels of health and well-being? How can these needs be measured?
- What alternative services are required to prevent the need for high-cost institutional placement? What are their costs and benefits? Are they cost-effective?
- Can financial and other incentives be developed to deliver the vast array of needed long-term care services in the most efficient and effective way?
- How can these medical and social long-term care services be financed in an equitable manner?
- What are the respective roles and responsibilities of the federal, state, and local governments, the community, private enterprise, and the individual in the delivery and financing of long-term care services?
- Can private insurance companies develop long-term care insurance plans that cover nursing home care, home health services, and social support services at a reasonable cost?
- Can the disparate elements that constitute the long-term care financing and delivery systems be brought together to fashion a coherent set of national policies on this important issue?

Policy issues in long-term care focus on four themes: the need for and use of long-term care; the determinants of such use; measures of need; and financing and reimbursement for long-term care. In a review of data needed to address these issues, certain key topics require priority attention: (1) how to define long-term care; (2) what data are required to understand and analyze the utilization of long-term care by the elderly; (3) how best to provide useful service statistics; and (4) how to collect, aggregate, and disseminate expenditure data.

DEFINITIONS OF LONG-TERM CARE

A major problem in assessing the magnitude of long-term care services and costs results from the lack of a common definition of long-term care in data collection and analysis. Both medical and nonmedical providers serve the long-term client. These providers may be public or private. Their services may be unique—the delivery of hot meals only, for example—or complex, as those provided in nursing homes or chronic disease hospitals. For many providers, their data systems, when such do exist, tend to be fragmented and incomplete.

Two definitions of long-term care are given here. The first is that used by the Health Care Financing Administration, the major federal agency dealing with payments for long-term care of the elderly; the second is that used in the Long-Term Health Care Minimum Data Set developed by the United States Committee on Vital and Health Statistics. Doty, Liu, and Weiner (1985), in an article in the *Health Care Financing Review*, state that "Long-term care (LTC) refers to health, social, and residential services provided to chronically disabled persons over an extended period of time." They go on to say, "the need for long-term care is not necessarily identified with particular diagnoses, but rather physical or mental disabilities that impair functioning in activities necessary for daily living" (Doty et al., 1985:69). In the introduction to the Long-Term Health Care Minimum Data Set, there is an expansion of the definition of long-term care: "Long term health care refers to the professional or personal services required on a recurring or continuous basis by an individual because of chronic or permanent physical or mental impairment. These services may be provided in a variety of settings including the client's own home" (U.S. Department of Health and Human Services, 1980b:31).

Each of the two definitions given above emphasizes two aspects of long-term care. First, it is care given over an extended period, and, second, the recipient of such care has lost some capacity for self-care due to chronic illness or condition, either physical or mental. Cure may not be a realistic goal in long-term care. The objectives of long-term care are to help persons to cope with their disabilities, to decrease their dependence on others, and to narrow the gap between their actual and potential function (U.S. Department of Health and Human Services, 1980b). The Minimum Data Set definition points out, in addition, that such care may be given in the person's own home. Family and community support may be as important to the person as medical care.

Essential to policy analysis is a common definition of long-term care. The ideal record system for long-term care should be capable of monitoring all necessary data on a person throughout the course of an illness regardless of where the care is received. The possibility of achieving such a record tracking system in the United States is unlikely. However, to the extent that all providers of care identify the care recipient in the same way and employ the same scales and classifications, their records can be assembled to answer questions as to client characteristics, long-term care usage, and the extent and nature of such service in relation to the intensity of care needed by the client.

>   **Recommendation 7.1:**   The panel recommends that the National Committee on Vital and Health Statistics develop a standard definition of long-term care for use by governmental and private programs emphasizing that it is care given over an extended time period and that the recipient of such care has lost some capacity for self-care.

UTILIZATION OF LONG-TERM CARE SERVICES BY THE ELDERLY

Service statistics and financial records may answer the question of who among the elderly uses long-term care. Unanswered, however, is the question of why some persons use long-term care services and others do not. The concept of functional disability has been developed in an attempt to describe the long-term care client. The elderly person's functional status is seen as an indicator of the services needed from the community. Diagnostic measures undertaken to determine appropriate levels of care have implications for resource allocation (German, 1981). The path by which persons become clients of long-term care services is less clearly understood. To trace this path through time is the goal of longitudinal studies. Improvement of the concept of functional disability and the introduction of longitudinal studies of the elderly will aid in understanding the utilization of long-term care.

Functional Disability

The diagnostic description of a person is seldom an indicator of his or her need for or utilization of long-term care because diagnosis alone gives no clue to how well or how poorly an individual functions. As a result, descriptions of behavior, rather than conditions, are used to describe the long-term care population. People in need of long-term care are commonly described as functionally limited or functionally disabled, those persons with a chronic physical or mental condition that impairs them so that they require the help of another person in performing everyday activities (Van Nostrand,

1985a). What constitutes functional limitation or functional disability, however, is still undecided. The federal Interagency Statistical Committee on Long-Term Care of Elderly (1980), in its effort to develop a definition of functional limitations, divided such limitations into four areas: mobility and transportation, personal care limitations, housekeeping limitations, and self-management limitations (Interagency Statistical Committee on Long-Term Care of the Elderly, 1980). In practice, however, most functional assessments of the elderly concentrate on only two areas: activities of daily living, which are personal care tasks, walking, bathing, dressing, eating, and toileting, and instrumental activities for daily living, which are selected tasks necessary for living independently in the community, such as shopping, preparing meals, doing household chores, managing money, using the telephone, and taking medicines (Van Nostrand, 1985b).

Missing from commonly used scales of ADL and IADL is any measure of either the behavior problems or the cognitive impairments that are frequently the cause of admission to long-term facilities. An individual still may be able to function physically and even to prepare some meals, yet be unable to avoid dangerous behavior such as crossing the street against the light or leaving the gas flame turned on. In the same way, cognitive impairments that result in an inability to identify familiar people or places may cause elderly individuals to wander and to lose their way. The Long-Term Health Care Minimum Data Set points out the importance of measures of behavior problems and of memory impairment in functional assessments of the elderly and also indicates the need for some measure of mood disturbance. The discussion of this topic states: "A persistent disturbance of mood is much more common in those with chronic medical conditions than in those who are physically healthy" (U.S. Department of Health and Human Services, 1980b:14).

The addition of measures of cognitive, social, and emotional functioning, including behavior problems and mood disturbances, to the current scales of functional disability would enhance the usefulness of such scales (see Katz et al., 1985). Including appropriate measures of these items in disability scales would improve the scales as predictive instruments both for the risk of institutionalization and for identifying heavy users of institutional services. Family members who may be able to deal with the physical problems of the elderly often find themselves unable to cope with behavior or cognitive problems or depression, turning to institutional care for their elderly relatives. A scale of functional disability enriched to include psychological and mental measures also would help to identify the heavy users of institutional services, since residents with such problems often require more care than those with chronic physical ailments only. A developmental phase would clearly be needed to resolve methodological issues in selecting effective measures. With the aging of the population, these problems assume increasing importance from many standpoints, including resource requirements, both public and private, and effects on family. While a standard set of measures poses methodological problems and has some cost consequences, the need is great. For example, the projected number of cases of severe dementia in the United States in the year 2000 is over 2 million (Cross and Gurland, 1986). In a study of Alzheimer's disease and other dementias the Office of Technology Assessment (1987) concluded that the exact costs of this type of illness to the nation cannot be calculated due to the paucity of relevant information, but it is clear that the annual cost is in billions of dollars.

> **Recommendation 7.2:** The panel recommends that the current national measures of functional disability be expanded by adding measures of cognitive, social, and emotional functioning, including behavior problems and mood disturbances, so that comparable information may be gathered from community and institutional populations.

The use of such measures would appear to be most relevant for supplements on aging in the NHIS, longitudinal studies on aging, and surveys of patients in nursing homes and other institutions.

Longitudinal Studies

Long-term care, by definition, is care over an extended time period. There are changes with time in the degree of impairment of older persons. Not all such changes are in a negative direction; people do improve as well as decline (Busse and Maddox, 1985). Residents are discharged from institutions not only to hospitals or to the funeral home but also to their own homes or to other community living arrangements. Aging is a process, and the transition points from health to disease need to be determined in both individuals and age cohorts. To project need for long-term care, data are required over a relatively long period (five or ten years) on the characteristics of the elderly population, their use of services, and the nature of their support system and changes in this system, both formal and informal.

Longitudinal studies of older persons must include both the well and the impaired in the community. The risk factors that may lead to institutionalization can be determined only through panel studies of both these groups, not by the descriptions and analyses of those persons admitted for institutional care, although such analyses may be useful for other purposes. Standardized definitions should be employed in describing community services and service providers, including the services given in the person's home.

Selected questions similar in content to those used in community studies should be used in longitudinal studies in institutions. Topics that need to be addressed include changes in health status, the outcome of care, and the costs of such care. Information on these topics from both the community elderly and those in institutions would make possible comparisons of the cost of care in different environments for elderly persons with comparable levels of disability.

Modifications and development of existing federal surveys could be used to develop the necessary data for studies of changes in health status and service utilization of the elderly over time. The 1982 and 1984 National Long-Term Care Surveys conducted by the Health Care Financing Administration and the Office of the Assistant Secretary of Health and the 1984 Supplement on Aging/National Health Interview Survey conducted by the National Center for Health Statistics are useful models for the development of longitudinal surveys of the aged in the community. The National Long-Term Care Surveys collected data on persons age 65 and older who were functionally disabled and living in the community. The sample was identified by telephone screening of persons in the Medicare health insurance enrollment file. Information was collected on degree of disability in cognitive functioning, the informal support system, the use of medical services, insurance coverage, and income. The 1982 Long-Term Care Survey also collected data about informal support given to elderly people. The 1984 survey was a follow-up of the 1982 survey, excluding the survey of informal supports but adding a sample of unimpaired people. A follow-up of the full 1984 sample, planned for 1988, should provide useful longitudinal information. The data for the disabled will be of particular interest since they will be data for a third point in time.

The 1984 Supplement on Aging of the National Health Interview Survey collected data on a sample of 8,000 persons age 55 and over in the community. In addition to information on health status and hospital and physician care, this survey collected information on income, housing, informal support, and the use of social services. A Social Security number was secured for each respondent to provide a future link with the National Death Index, so that cause of death could be linked with previously collected information (Van Nostrand, 1985a). With the cooperation of and funding from the National Institute on Aging, persons who were age 70 and over in 1984 were reinterviewed in 1987. The usefulness of these materials for longitudinal analysis would be greatly enhanced if data were collected for all persons in the 1984 survey, beginning with those age 55 and older.

> **Recommendation 7.3:** The panel recommends that the National Center on Health Statistics continue to collect, every two years, health and other relevant information (hospital and physician care, income, housing, informal support, and the use of community services) from all persons age 55 and older in the original sample of persons in the 1984 Supplement on Aging of the National Health Interview Survey, now known as the Longitudinal Study on Aging.

The National Nursing Home Survey conducted by the National Center for Health Statistics in 1977 and 1985 is a useful model for longitudinal surveys of the institutional elderly. These surveys collected data on the characteristics of the nursing home, its costs, and its staff, as well as on the characteristics of both current residents and discharged patients. For the 1985 survey, the center is conducting a follow-up of residents and discharged patients.

Information collected for both current residents and discharged patients includes functional disability, chronic conditions, services received, charges for care, and sources of payment. Data on discharges includes the duration of stay and its outcome. The 1985 survey also collected data from next of kin of both residents and discharged patients on functional disability at time of admission, caregiver stress, and the family's view of the reasons for admission. Items on functional disability in both surveys were structured so that they were similar to data on functional disability in community samples. Like the 1984 SOA/NHIS, the 1985 NNHS collected Social Security numbers for matching to the National Death Index (Van Nostrand, 1985b).

> **Recommendation 7.4:** The panel recommends that the National Nursing Home Survey (a) be conducted on a 3-5 year

cycle, (b) be expanded to include all types of long-term care institutions (i.e., chronic disease hospitals, mental health facilities, rehabilitation centers, board and care homes, psychiatric halfway houses, and residential facilities), and (c) that a subsample of admission cohorts in the 1985 survey serve as a panel for a longitudinal study of institutionalized persons and that the records of the subsample be linked with Medicare files.

Other important longitudinal surveys are the NHANES Epidemiologic Follow-up Survey, discussed in Chapter 3, and the EPESE study, discussed in Chapter 1.

SERVICE STATISTICS

Long-term care services include a broad continuum of health care, social services, and residential care. These services are provided in settings that are either institution- or community-based. All of these service providers collect some statistical data for administrative bodies—federal, state, and local. The conflicting and overlapping demands on providers of services by funding and regulatory agencies are a serious burden to limited staff. Evaluation of aspects of care in different settings can scarcely be accomplished without special studies (Murnaghan, 1976). The collection of uniform or standard data relating to long-term care by service agencies would yield comparable information on providers of care, services given, and the characteristics of the long-term care population. Special problems relevant to the collection of service statistics are considered here.

Providers of Care

Long-term care for the elderly is delivered in health facilities such as nursing homes, chronic disease hospitals, mental health facilities, and rehabilitation centers; in housing with support services, such as board and care homes, life-care communities, psychiatric halfway houses, and residential facilities; by home-health and other agencies in the client's own home; and by social service agencies providing adult day care, income maintenance, home-delivered meals, and transportation, among other services. Inventories are available of nursing homes, psychiatric facilities, and Medicare- or Medicaid-certified providers. There are no comprehensive inventories of currently unlisted health and social facilities such as board and care homes and home health agencies. In order to manage or monitor health care and health-related services, agencies, and institutions, the definition of long-term care providers should be expanded to include community services for the long-term client, both medical and nonmedical.

Recommendation 7.5: The panel recommends that the National Master Facility Inventory compiled by the National Center for Health Statistics from census data and state records be expanded to cover all health and social facilities providing long-term care. In addition to providers currently listed, the expansion would include board and care homes, home health agencies, and adult day-care centers.

There has been an enormous expansion in residential facilities for the elderly, many of which provide long-term care and support services. Such residential facilities include retirement homes, shared living arrangements, board and care homes, and others. A sampling frame is needed for the study of such facilities; this would entail the development of definitions that distinguish among the various types of housing providing support services and between housing and health care institutions as defined by the National Master Facility Inventory (NMFI). The decennial census is an important resource in this area. The Bureau of the Census included a question that separately identified board and care facilities and the types of care they provide in the national content pretest, which will be used to develop the final content of the 1990 census. Board and care housing was defined as the provision by a nonrelative of food, shelter, and some degree of protective oversight or personal care that is generally nonmedical in nature. Because the quality of the pretest data from the board and care housing question could not be determined, the question will not be included in the 1990 census. The response burden of the board and care question is so large that it is unlikely that it would be included in any census. With the goal of developing a nationwide list of board and care facilities, the Bureau of the Census and the Department of Health and Human Services should be encouraged to explore ways to identify such facilities by building on the 1990 census. One approach would be to do a follow-up study of households with three or more unrelated adults in the 1990 census.

Types of Care

A standard classification of the types of care given by long-term providers is essential. Only in this way can data be made available to evaluate the quality and effectiveness of services provided in different environments and by various health care professionals. A classification of a broad range of services is given in the Long-Term Health Care Minimum Data Set. This classification, or some modification of it, can be used for reporting purposes by different types of providers who are giving the same or similar care to the elderly.

Recommendation 7.6: The panel recommends that the National Committee on Vital and Health Statistics evaluate and, if necessary, revise the Long-Term Health Care Minimum Data Set's classification of types of services given by providers of long-term care.

Informal Supports

National surveys indicate that there are twice as many elderly persons bedfast and housebound at home as there are in institutions of all kinds (Shanas, 1982). These long-term patients living at home are given care by family, friends, and neighbors as well as by members of formally organized service organizations. The care given by family, friends, and neighbors is usually described as informal support. There is need for standard definitions of informal and formal support. Is care given in the household by a practical nurse who is not affiliated with an organization but whose salary is paid by a family member informal support? Definitions of informal support need to distinguish between support given by family members both inside and outside the household, and that given by household members whether or not relatives of the recipient. These distinctions may well be significant in terms of the stability and intensity of support received by the elderly. A particularly vulnerable group are elderly people living alone. The lack of clear definitions in types of informal support creates ambiguities and leads to misinterpretation of data.

More information is needed about the providers of informal care. The spouse and children of the elderly person are the major caregivers of functionally limited old people at home. There is no clear marker for when, and at what point, the providers of informal care call on formal support as either a care supplement or as a replacement of their services. Are the people taken care of through informal support less impaired than those receiving formal support? Can one type of caregiver replace another? The relationship between the giving of informal care and the degree of impairment of the recipient needs investigation.

The need for this type of information was recognized in planning the 1982 National Long-Term Care Survey, which included a special component on caregivers who provide assistance to the elderly with the activities of daily living. Data were collected on the characteristics of the caregiver, including assistance provided, associated stress, and opportunity costs (i.e., the cost to the caregiver of opportunities foregone because of time spent in providing care.) The cross-sectional data from this survey and the 1984 Supplement on Aging of the National Health Interview Study both have provided important information about informal support (Van Nostrand, 1985a). However, changes are needed to meet requirements for data on caretakers for future development of policies on services for the elderly.

> **Recommendation 7.7:** The panel recommends that (a) the National Committee on Vital and Health Statistics develop a standard definition of informal supports that distinguishes between family members and nonfamily members (i.e., friends and neighbors) and identifies whether the helping individual lives in the same household as the care recipient and (b) that information on caretakers be an integral part of cross-sectional surveys and longitudinal studies of the elderly in the community.

In addition, information is needed about the availability of the informal caretakers of the elderly currently and in the future. Most family caretakers, spouses or adult children, are women. Adult female children of the elderly are likely to be less available as caretakers in the future as a result of changes in family size, increasing employment among middle-aged women, and physical distance from elderly parents. Models have been proposed for forecasting the informal support networks of the future elderly that address demographic variables (i.e., marriages, births, divorces, labor force participation) and relate these to health status and disability of the elderly (Manton and Soldo, 1985; Myers, 1985).

STANDARDIZATION OF MINIMUM DATA SETS

The Long-Term Health Care Minimum Data Set developed by the National Committee on Vital and Health Statistics includes data items about clients, services, and costs. The data set defines the central core of information about the long-term care client needed on a routine basis by most users and establishes standard measurements, definitions, and classifications for this core (U.S. Department of Health and Human Services, 1980b). Work on the data set began at a conference in 1975 in which a representative, multidisciplinary group of providers and users of information on long-term care discussed the characteristics of such care, the data requirements of different users, and methods of measurement, and data collection and presentation. The appointment of a Technical Consultant Panel on Long-Term Care followed this conference. Representatives from virtually all government agencies and bureaus concerned with long-term care, as well as a number of outside experts, participated in the work of the panel.

The data set was circulated in draft form for comment to a large group of potential users and interested organizations including planning agencies, state officials, third-party payers, and professional organizations (U.S. Department of Health and Human Services, 1980b). In final form the data set was also evaluated by a representative group of users. It has been adapted for use in the extended care program of the Veterans Administration.

Surveys and administrative records in long-term care need uniform definitions of the same topic. Without such definitions, data gathered by one source cannot be compared or aggregated with data gathered by another. The data set, as developed, permits flexibility in health information systems without the loss of the ability to make basic comparisons. General use of the data set would open the door to developing comparable information from different sources on the providers of care, services given, and health status and demographic characteristics of the service recipient. Potential applications of the data set include: (1) management or monitoring of health and health-related services, agencies and institutions, (2) management of care of patients and service clients, and (3) allocation of resources to agencies and programs. The Long-Term Health Care Minimum Data Set is currently undergoing the usual Department of Health and Human Services administrative and policy review process prior to implementation.

Recommendation 7.8: The panel recommends the use of the Long-Term Health Care Minimum Data Set by the Health Care Financing Administration, the National Center for Health Statistics, the Bureau of the Census, and other federal agencies in appropriate long-term care administrative, survey, and research data collection activities. The data set should be periodically reviewed by the National Committee on Vital and Health Statistics in light of changes in health delivery systems and public policy.

For example, nursing homes could incorporate the data set in their administrative records (the Veterans Administration is already doing so), the Health Care Financing Administration could include a requirement for use of the data set when they issue requests for research proposals on long-term care, and the National Center for Health Statistics could adopt the data set in the LSOA and the NNHS.

EXPENDITURE DATA ON LONG-TERM CARE

With the projected growth of the older population, particularly of the very old among them, the demand for long-term care may be expected to increase. National expenditures for long-term care may also be expected to increase. Most of the national expenditures for long-term care are for nursing home or institutional care, although expenditures for noninstitutional care also have increased rapidly (Doty et al., 1985).

Estimates of nursing home care are part of the National Health Expenditure series, which was initiated in the Department of Health, Education, and Welfare and is currently prepared and published each fall by the Health Care Financing Administration. Most of this care is provided to elderly people. In 1985, $35.2 billion, almost 1 percent of the gross national producet, went for nursing home care (Waldo et al., 1986). Only $0.6 billion of this amount came from Medicare funds (the Veterans' Administration paid a similar amount, $0.7 billion). Patients and their families accounted for $18.1 billion (private insurance and other private funds for $0.6 billion); Medicaid paid $14.7 billion.

Home health care is a growing segment of the health care delivery system. Expenditures for these services are not broken out separately in the National Health Expenditure series but are included under "other professional services" along with services such as podiatric care (Van Nostrand, 1985b). Nevertheless, Medicare spending for home health care is estimated to have grown from $60 million in 1968 to $2.3 billion in 1985 (Waldo et al., 1986).

Additional long-term care services for the elderly are not reported in the National Health Expenditure series. Among such services are the costs of social services funded by states through social service block grants, and services funded through the Older Americans Act and other federal programs. The National Medical Expenditure Survey planned for 1987 will collect information on health status of individuals, their medical cost expenditures, and the source of payment for the civilian population as well as for the population in nursing homes, psychiatric hospitals, and facilities for the mentally retarded. The aggregation of these data from both households and institutions will provide an overview of expenditures for long-term care. These data, together with the data reported under public programs, will provide a basis for the development of an ongoing series on expenditures for long-term care, which accounts for a large and growing proportion of public and private health care expenditures. These data are essential for estimating the costs of alternative policies for the provision of long-term care.

Recommendation 7.9: The panel recommends that aggregate national expenditure data for long-term care of the elderly, including expenditures for both health and social services, be prepared and disseminated by the Health Care Financing Administration using as a model the National Health Accounts.

8
The Financing of Health Care Services for the Elderly

INTRODUCTION

Spending on health care services for the elderly has been increasing since 1965; between 1977 and 1984 it increased at an annual rate of 14.5 percent (Waldo and Lazenby, 1984). The increase in expenditures is reflected in the increasing cost to the federal and state governments of operating the Medicare and Medicaid programs as well as in the increase in out-of-pocket payments made by the elderly. As a consequence, health care financing has become one of the more critical policy issues to be addressed by the nation.

The methods used to finance health care services have important effects on the use of health care services by the elderly and their level of health and well being, as well as on the growth and development of the health care sector itself. In addition, the methods used to finance health care services influence the distribution of income between the sick and the well, the old and the young, the general taxpayer and the recipients of care.

Many types of data are required to provide a factual basis for policy issues related to the financing of health care services for an aging population. Although a policy issue is seldom resolved by using only data from a national information system, such data are frequently used to address some elements of a policy issue. For example, in the list of policy issues that follows, the first would probably require an evaluation study, but Medicare records could provide historical information on the cost of the fee-for-service systems and the HMOs.

To address the second issue, data from the National Medical Expenditure Survey could be used to identify the most costly of the various chronic illnesses and help to limit the illnesses to be addressed by the policy analyst. Selected emerging policy questions that need to be addressed follow:

- Will health maintenance organizations, social health maintenance organizations (SHMOs), and preferred provider organizations (PPOs) serve as less costly alternatives to the current fee-for-service system?
- How can we control expenditures for health and long-term care in the face of the projected growth of the elderly who are at risk of chronic illness often requiring extensive medical and long-term care services? Will people have to do without medical care?
- What aspects of the growing health needs of an aging society are most affected by the pressures to constrain budgetary and economic resources devoted to health care?
- What mechanisms are needed to share the burden of health care expenditures for an aging society more equitably among all members of society?
- What is the impact of the Medicare prospective payment system based on diagnosis-related groups on providers, patients, expenditures, and access to and quality of care?
- With the growing financial burden of out-of-pocket expenditures for certain groups of the elderly who are disabled and require extensive treatment, what are the alternative equitable financing mechanisms to pay for these services?
- What alternative financing mechanisms for the supply of long-term care services should be supported and by whom?
- What changes in funding mechanisms, legislation, and public policy are necessary to shift the emphasis away from hospital and nursing home care toward less costly alternatives?
- Can less costly and less restrictive alternative services to institutionalization be developed to maintain the independence of the elderly? Can economic incentives be developed for in-home and community-based services to maintain the elderly at home?
- What is the viability of tax credits, reverse mortgages, independent retirement accounts, and the like in assisting the elderly to pay for a greater share of their health and long-term care costs? Are there other private-sector alternatives?

- What are the costs (direct and indirect) of chronic illnesses such as Alzheimer's disease and what are the implications of helping to meet those costs through public funding?
- To what extent is there an emerging intergenerational inequity with the aging of the baby boom generation—Americans born between 1946 and 1964—and low fertility rates in which a smaller number of the working population will bear the burden of support of the larger number of retired elderly beginning about the year 2010?

This section of the report focuses on specific aspects of the financing of health care services for the elderly population. First, it describes the major public programs that cover health care services for the aged as well as the other sources of funding for health care. Since many of these programs are undergoing significant changes, the direction of that change is outlined. Next it presents information on the level of expenditures and source of payment by type of service for the aged, including the distribution of expenditures across the aged population. Data needs and recommendations are presented with reference to the policy issues emerging from the current proposed changes in financing mechanisms.

Sources of Funding

In describing the current methods of financing care for the elderly, it is appropriate to begin with a brief description of the public programs, in particular Medicare and Medicaid. These are the most important sources of funding, and the structure of these program affects the nature of the insurance policies that are offered by the private sector.

Medicare

Approximately 95 percent of all people age 65 and over in the United States are covered by the Medicare program. Medicare consists of two separate but complementary programs: Hospital Insurance (HI) for services furnished in hospitals, in skilled nursing facilities, and by home health agencies; and Supplementary Medical Insurance (SMI) for the services of physicians, home health visits (for people who may not be covered by HI), outpatient services, and the costs of durable medical equipment and prostheses. Coverage for outpatient mental health services is very restricted. In addition, some services frequently used by the elderly, such as outpatient drugs, dental services, and eyeglasses, are not covered.

The Medicare program was explicitly designed to cover the major costs associated with episodes of acute illness or the acute manifestations of chronic illness. The extent to which the program actually pays for services such as skilled nursing facilities and home health, usually considered long-term care services is therefore very limited.

People are automatically enrolled in HI within a short time of reaching their sixty-fifth birthday. The costs of HI are covered by Social Security payroll taxes paid into a trust fund by employers and employees. Enrollment in SMI is contingent on paying a premium that covers about 25 percent of the cost. There is some beneficiary cost sharing on Medicare-covered services. The cost-sharing provisions were included in the original legislation both to control federal budget expenditures as well as to deter unnecessary utilization. The actual cost-sharing provisions are complicated and vary from service to service.

When Medicare was first enacted, the Congress incorporated into the program many of the standard features of the Blue Cross/Blue Shield plans that were then the dominant form of private health insurance. The most important features were beneficiary freedom of choice of providers, cost-based reimbursement of institutional providers, and fee-for-service reimbursements based on reasonable charges for physicians' services. With the exception of long-term care services, there were few limitations placed on the use of covered services. There were no incentives for hospitals to control costs and no rewards for improving efficiency. The reimbursement provisions are currently undergoing major changes. In 1982, changes were made in the law to stimulate the enrollment of Medicare recipients into prepaid group practices; in 1983 the cost-based reimbursement system for hospitals was replaced with a prospective payment system under which hospitals are paid a fixed amount for taking care of patients based on their discharge diagnosis. In 1985 the Reagan administration proposed replacing the current physician reimbursement system with a fee schedule. The federal government is also evaluating ways for bringing other providers of care under prospective payment (Davis and Rowland, 1986:Chapter 3).

Between 1977 and 1984, payments for services under Medicare increased at an annual rate of 17.3 percent per year. By 1984 Medicare expenditures for the elderly amounted to $58.5 billion, making it the third largest federal program (Waldo and Lazenby, 1984). As a result of the rapid escalation in the cost of the program, the reimbursement changes outlined above were made. In addition to those changes, the administration and Congress are seeking other ways of lowering the costs of the program, such as increasing the cost-sharing requirements, changing the age for eligibility, increasing the premium costs, making Medicare the second payer for those who are employed and eligible for employer-provided health insurance, increasing Medicare enrollment in HMOs, and changing the Medicare program to a voucher program. (This description of the Medicare program and the following discussion of Medicaid are based heavily on Sawyer et al., 1983.)

Medicaid

Medicaid, a program to provide medical services to the poor, is administered by the states under federal guidelines. With respect to the elderly, Medicaid pays for the medical care for those who meet Supplementary Security Income (SSI) standards. States have the option of covering medically needy individuals (those with incomes slightly above the SSI levels) and individuals who have incurred sufficiently high medical expenditures that they "spend down" to Medicaid income eligibility levels.

For dually eligible recipients, Medicare is the first payer for Medicare-covered services and Medicaid is the second payer; that is, Medicaid will pay the cost-sharing amounts that would normally fall to the patient. Depending on the state's program, Medicaid may also pay for the cost of services not covered by Medicare, such as outpatient, drug, optical, and dental services. More important, as Medicare fulfilled its purpose of covering most of the costs related to acute episodes, Medicaid has evolved into the primary public funding source for long-term services for the elderly.

Like the Medicare program, the costs of the Medicaid program have been increasing at a rapid rate. Between 1977 and 1984, Medicaid expenditures on behalf of the elderly increased at an annual rate of 14.2 percent—largely due to coverage of nursing home care. In 1984, expenditures for the population age 65 and over were approximately $12.8 billion (Waldo and Lazenby, 1984). As with Medicare, there is a concerted effort to reevaluate the structure of the program, in particular with respect to long-term services, to revise the methods used to reimburse providers, especially nursing homes, and to change the income eligibility levels.

The Veterans Administration

Until recently, all veterans age 65 years and over were eligible for Veterans Administration (VA) services. A recent law made several changes in a veteran's eligibility for VA health care regardless of age, which became effective July 1, 1986. Actual access to health care services is now determined through an eligibility assessment, with first priority being given to veterans with service-connected disabilities or to those who meet a means test known as the category A means test. These veterans are eligible for hospital care in VA facilities. Outpatient and nursing home care may be provided in VA facilities if space is available. Veterans with nonservice-connected disabilities and with income above the category A means test but below a higher level, known as the category B means test, may receive hospital, outpatient, and nursing home care in VA facilities if space is available. Veterans with nonservice-connected disabilities and with income above the category B means test may receive VA services if space is available, but they must agree to pay a deductible amount for care equivalent to the payment that would be required by Medicare. In addition to the VA-owned and operated facilities, which include hospitals and their associated outpatient departments and nursing homes, the Veterans Administration contracts for skilled and intermediate care at community nursing homes on a per diem basis. However, with the exception of care provided to veterans with service-connected disabilities, the VA will not pay for more than 6 months of care in community facilities. In 1984, $3.3 billion was spent for health care of aged veterans.

The actual use of the VA system by elderly veterans is contingent on the characteristics of the elderly that define eligibility, the availability of VA-owned facilities, and the access to the private sector by VA eligibles. Since most veterans are covered by Medicare, the service that is likely to be most attractive to the older veteran is nursing home care. However, the main factor that will influence the veteran's use of nursing home services is the number of nursing home beds available within the VA system. Before July 1986, approximately 10 to 12 percent of elderly veterans actually used the system (U.S. Congressional Budget Office, 1984). This number may change as a result of the current and proposed changes in Medicare and the new eligibility procedures for VA health care.

Other Government Programs

There are a number of other programs that have been developed to finance health care expenditures for the elderly. Included are the Department of Defense Civilian Health and Medical Program of the Uniformed Services, which provides care for active and retired military forces and their dependents, state and local government hospitals providing community and psychiatric hospital services to older citizens, federal grant programs, and state and local public assistance programs providing services that are not eligible for federal matching funds under the Medicaid program. In 1984, a total of $3.4 billion was spent for the elderly by government programs other than Medicare, Medicaid, and the VA.

Private Insurance Programs

There are a number of private insurance policies that have been specifically designed for the elderly. In general, most of these policies fill the gaps in Medicare-covered services, such as the coinsurance and deductible provisions, rather than extending insurance protection against uncovered services such as long-term care services or outpatient drugs (Rice and McCall, 1985). With the projected large increase in the number of people age 65 and over, especially those age 85 and over, there is increased interest in finding mechanisms for stimulating the development of private insurance coverage for long-term care services (Meiners, 1985a).

Of the noninstitutionalized elderly, approximately 65 percent have private policies that supplement Medicare, 10 percent are covered by Medicaid, 20 percent are covered by Medicare only, and 4 percent had some other form of coverage (Garfinkel and Corder, 1984). Among the elderly not eligible for Medicaid, those who are better educated, have higher incomes, and are in slightly better health are more likely to purchase a supplemental health insurance policy.

Expenditures on Health Care

In 1984, personal health care expenditures for the elderly amounted to $119.9 billion, or $4,202 per person age 65 and over (Waldo and Lazenby, 1984). Of this total, 25.2 percent was paid by the consumer directly, 7.2 percent through private insurance, 48.8 percent by Medicare, 12.8 percent by Medicaid, and 5.6 percent by

TABLE 8.1 Health Care Expenditures for the Noninstitutionalized Elderly, 1980 (percentage)

Health Care Expenditures	Proportion of Noninstitutionalized Elderly	Proportion of Expenditures
Less than $500	60	6
$500-$3,000	26	19
Over $3,000	14	75

Source: Kovar (1986).

other government programs, primarily the Veterans Administration. However, these averages mask the wide differences in the funding sources for different types of medical services. The extremes are represented by sources of expenditures on hospitals and nursing homes. In 1984, hospital expenditures for the elderly amounted to $54.9 billion ($1,900 per capita) of which 3.1 percent was paid by the patient directly, 7.9 percent through private insurance, 74.8 percent by Medicare, 4.8 percent by Medicaid, and 9.1 percent by other government programs. Nursing home expenditures in the same year amounted to $25.1 billion ($880 per capita), of which 50.1 percent was paid for by the patient directly, 1.1 percent by private insurance, 2.1 percent by Medicare, 41.5 percent by Medicaid, and 4.4 percent by other government programs (Waldo and Lazenby, 1984).

Since the elderly population is heterogeneous, average expenditures provide an incomplete picture of the cost of illness and the sources of funding. For example, consider the 1980 National Medical Care Utilization and Expenditure Survey expenditures data for three groups of the noninstitutionalized elderly: the "low-cost" users, those with expenditures less than $500, "medium-cost" users, with expenditures between $500 and $3,000, and the "high-cost" users, those with expenditures over $3,000. Although these categories are somewhat arbitrary, they help to establish the well-known fact that health care expenditures are concentrated on a small number of sick people. As shown in Table 8.1, only 14 percent of the noninstitutionalized elderly had health care expenditures over $3,000, but they accounted for 75 percent of total expenditure of health care services made on behalf of the elderly.

Five percent of the elderly in the survey were institutionalized or died during 1980. Expenditures for this group emphasize even more strikingly the concentration of dollar costs for the seriously ill. During the part of the year that these persons were in the community, they accounted for 22 percent of the total health care expenditures for the elderly.

As noted earlier, the share of expenditures paid directly by the consumer also varied by the nature of the health care received. Elderly persons who were not hospitalized paid, on average, 67 percent of their medical care charges, while the elderly who had been hospitalized paid 18 percent. Because the total hospital charges are high, this out-of-pocket charge for the hospitalized group was about $650, while the nonhospitalized paid $202 (Kovar, 1986). It should be stressed, moreover, that these numbers conceal differences in out-of-pocket liability for the institutionalized population. People in nursing homes, who incur large out-of-pocket expenditures—because both the cost of the service is so high and insurance is so limited—are not included in the National Medical Care Utilization and Expenditure Survey, the source of the above data.

The Frail Elderly

One group of elderly that is receiving considerable attention are those with potential needs for long-term care services—the frail and dependent elderly. In 1982 approximately 19 percent of the elderly age 65 and over (4.6 million people) needed help in activities of daily living or in instrumental activities of daily living, and the size of this group will increase with the aging of the population (Liu et al., 1985). We actually know very little about the total cost of care for this population: they represent such a small part of the general population that they have not been adequately represented in national household surveys (such as the 1977 National Medical Care Expenditure Survey and the 1980 National Medical Care Utilization and Expenditure Survey), the major sources of information on the distribution of health care services across the aged population.

This group is of particular interest because there is currently limited public and private insurance to help them meet the cost of long-term care services and because it is believed that fostering home-based care may offer a cost-effective alternative to nursing home care. Thus, one major health financing issue is the extent to which public insurance programs should support home-based programs.

This is a very complicated issue because most of the home care services received by this group of people are provided by family members or by members of the helping organizations. In fact, approximately 72 percent of the services rendered are provided by family members (Liu et al., 1985). Although the use of formal (i.e., paid for) services increases with the level of disability, 65 percent of people with many limitations in activities of daily living relied solely on informal care (Liu et al., 1985). The current extensive use of unpaid health care makes it very difficult to design a public financing program for health care services that will encourage the efficient substitution of home-based services for nursing home services, because any such program is also likely to lead to a substitution of services provided by the family or already paid for by the individuals or their families for publicly funded home care services.

Thus in evaluating proposals to change the financing of long-term care services for the elderly, data are needed to assess the extent that financing mechanisms will lead to an increase in the use of services or to a substitution of publicly funded services for services previously provided by the family free of charge or paid by the individuals and their families. If new services are used, to what extent will they act as complements or as substitutes for nursing home care? In addition, what is the effect of the use of new services on the health status of the elderly, to what extent do these services lead to an increase in their quality of life, and what is the effect of this new financing on the proportion of the family's income that is spent on health care?

Future Changes

All aspects of health care financing programs are currently being reevaluated: program eligibility, in particular the extent to which income and assets should determine access to public programs; appropriate roles of public versus private sources of funding; the scope of the covered services, appropriate levels of beneficiary cost sharing; the level and basis of payments to providers; the level of quality of care that should be guaranteed by public funds; and the types of services to be promoted by public funds.

As the organization, delivery, and financing of medical care services are changed, we need data that will allow us to address the following questions: How do the changes affect the cost of care, the distribution of the burden of paying for the care across public and private sources of funding and among individuals, and the health status and quality of life of the elderly?

DATA REQUIREMENTS

In order to develop and guide policy for financing health care for the elderly and to monitor the impact of changes in such financing, it is necessary to have a variety of data, including person-based survey data, administrative record data, and actuarial data. Survey data should include information on health status, income, assets, medical care expenditures, and sources of payment for medical care. Data need to be sufficiently detailed so that reliable statistics can be created for the most vulnerable of the elderly—the frail elderly, low-income elderly, and minorities. This information should be collected on both people residing in institutions and people living in the community.

Additional data that are useful in the analysis of financing medical care services are the administrative records of the Health Care Financing Administration, the Social Security Administration and the Internal Revenue Service. These data are by-products of administering large programs, and their statistical systems are reasonably inexpensive. There are two major constraints impeding the usefulness of these data for policy purposes. The first is that the agencies do not have adequate staffs to analyze the data, a fact that results in significant lags in the production of data and analyses. This problem is likely to become more acute over time. The second is that there are many restrictions imposed on making public use of data tapes, a subject that is discussed in more detail in Chapter 11.

Actuarial data from private insurers are also needed for establishing the costs of alternative long-term care policies. Minimal data are available on costs and utilization of long-term care insurance, and very little of the data reflects actual experience. A further complicating factor is that private insurers are reluctant to share their limited data bases to enable the development and marketing of long-term care insurance. Although the number of companies providing long-term care insurance is growing, there is also active discussion of federal coverage of long-term care costs for the population not covered by Medicaid.

Timely Data on Expenditures for the Elderly

The Health Care Financing Administration periodically publishes data on health care expenditures of the population age 65 and over by type of expenditure and source of funds. These data are estimated from secondary sources, including administrative records of the Medicare and Medicaid programs and surveys conducted by NCHS, HCFA, and NCHSR. Health expenditures of the elderly population are part of the national health expenditure accounts for the entire population published annually by HCFA.

National health expenditure data are widely used by policy makers to evaluate the extent of coverage of existing public programs, such as Medicare and Medicaid, of the total health care costs of the elderly population. They also serve as a basis for assessing the possible consequences of changes in public policy and programs, although this is always a question of the relevance of current and past data to a possible future program that changes the eligibility rules of current or past programs. For example, current cost and utilization data reflect the effects of the current mix of private and public insurance for the elderly. Changes in policy regarding long-term care financing would alter the situation, and it is important in the development of data to consider requirements to provide reasonable estimates of these effects.

Because of the policy uses of these aggregate expenditures data for the elderly population by source of funds and type of expenditures, their publication on a regular basis is important.

> **Recommendation 8.1:** The panel recommends that the Health Care Financing Administration develop and publish timely annual estimates of the national health expenditures by age. These estimates should follow the publication of the estimates of expenditures for the total population by a few months at most. At a minimum, these health expenditures for the population age 65 and over should include estimates by type of expenditure and source of funds and by age (ages 65-74, ages 75-84, and age 85 and over).

National Medical Expenditure Survey

The 1987 National Medical Expenditure Survey follows a series of national medical expenditures surveys, including the 1980 National Medical Care Utilization and Expenditures Survey and the 1977 National Medical Care Expenditures Survey.

Like the NMCES and the NMCUES, the NMES surveys a national probability sample of the civilian noninstitutionalized population. The NMES Household Survey is a year-long panel collecting measures of health status, use of health care services, expenditures and sources of payment, insurance coverage, employment, income and assets, and demographic information. When information planned for collection is the same as that collected for the NMCES and the NMCUES, and the previously used questions were found satisfactory, the same wording was retained. A particular focus is community-based long-term care. Household data are supplemented by surveys of medical and health insurance providers and by data from Medicare administrative files. In planning for future surveys, the panel urges the National Center for Health Services Research and Health Care Technology to continue this policy of providing comparability of data items between surveys.

A major gap in the NMCES and the NMCUES is the lack of data for the institutionalized population. Since at least 85 percent of the institutionalized population is age 65 and over, the omission of expenditures for this population group presented serious gaps in accurately estimating the health care costs of the elderly population. An important feature of the NMES is an Institutional Population Component (IPC), which will survey about 10,000 persons in nursing homes, facilities for the mentally retarded, and psychiatric hospitals and collect data similar to those for the noninstitutionalized household population. The IPC universe includes all persons in these long-term care institutions for any part of 1987. IPC and household data will provide the first composite picture of the nation's use of long-term health care.

The institutional component will permit analysis of long-term care for the nation, including special attention to the increasing number in the age groups 75 and older. Current plans include the incorporation into the data base of three groups of providers of long-term institutional care: nursing homes, facilities for the mentally retarded, and psychiatric hospitals. Each of these types of facilities provides care to substantial numbers of federal beneficiaries, primarily Medicaid recipients.

With this institutional component, the analytic potential of the NMES will encompass national estimates of health services use, expenditures, and insurance coverage for: (1) the entire U.S. civilian population, including the institutionalized; (2) the entire long-term care population, whether residing in institutions or in the community; and (3) institutionalized groups of persons in nursing homes, facilities for the mentally retarded, and psychiatric hospitals.

The current sample design for the National Medical Expenditure Survey, as the panel understands it, will provide reliable estimates for two age groups, 65-74 and 75 and over. However, since the group age 85 and over is the most rapidly growing segment of the population and the group that makes the greatest use of health care services, it will be critically important to collect information on their use of health care service.

> **Recommendation 8.2:** The panel recommends that the sample of the elderly population for the household survey for future national medical expenditure surveys be large enough to provide accurate estimates to study utilization and expenditures for medical care for three elderly age groups: 65-74, 75-84, and 85 and over.

The National Medical Expenditure Survey will provide a rich source of data on the health services utilization and expenditure patterns of the community-residing and institutionalized elderly. Its panel design may permit assessment of the impact of changes in service delivery and payment systems experienced by some of its respondents during the course of a calendar year on their utilization of health services and expenditures for health care. In addition, the planned linkage between the survey data collected during this year-long panel and the Medicare records of those persons age 65 and over in the samples should enhance the value of the utilization and expenditure data collected. However, to capture trends in utilization and expenditure patterns in response to changes in delivery and payment systems over time, a national medical care expenditure survey should be conducted periodically. These data are used for estimating the cost of policy alternatives for health care—policy uses that require more recent data than those currently available. In addition, changes in health care expenditures and utilization stimulate policy questions that affect decisions about public financing and regulation of services.

> **Recommendation 8.3:** The panel recommends that a national medical care expenditure survey be conducted periodically. The periodicity should be determined in relation to policy needs and the timing of other health-related surveys.

The NMES survey should be a joint effort of appropriate federal agencies (including the National Center for Health Services Research and Health Care Technology, the Health Care Financing Administration, and the National Center for Health Statistics) in order to take full advantage of the various types of relevant expertise in those agencies.

Follow-up Studies of the Elderly in the NMES through Administrative Records

A major gap in understanding the impact of changes in financing of medical care services in individuals and their families is the lack of longitudinal data on the use of and expenditures for medical care services as a person ages and is at risk of chronic illness requiring acute medical and long-term care services.

A considerable amount of data about the sampled individuals is also available from administrative records of HCFA, SSA, and IRS. The National Death Index conducted by NCHS also provides information on an individual's death. This rich source of information from administrative records can enhance the usefulness of the survey data collected in the NMES for longitudinal analyses at minimum costs.

> **Recommendation 8.4:**　The panel recommends that the National Center for Health Services Research and Health Care Technology identify and follow the population age 55 and over in the 1987 National Medical Expenditure Survey through the linking of administrative records, including Medicare reimbursements from Health Care Financing Administration records, and, to the extent feasible, Medicaid reimbursements from state record systems. In addition, the National Death Index of the Center for Health Statistics should be used to identify the year and cause of death of each sampled person.

In carrying out these record linkages, it would be essential that NCHSR comply with confidentiality restrictions.

Outreach Program for the NMES and Timely Release of NMES Tapes

The analytic potential of the NMES encompasses national estimates of health services use, expenditures, and insurance coverage. These data must be shared in a timely fashion with the researchers in the academic and private sectors as well as researchers in other government agencies, many of whom are directly involved with policy makers.

Several federal agencies, including the National Center for Health Statistics and the Census Bureau, have been successful in assisting outside researchers in the efficient use of their public use data tapes by conducting conferences for data tape users throughout the country.

Recommendation 8.5: The panel recommends that the National Center for Health Services Research and the Health Care Financing Administration: (a) begin planning an outreach program, including the conduct of conferences for data tape users similar to those conducted by federal agencies such as the National Center for Health Statistics and the Census Bureau, to inform and educate the policy and research communities in the efficient use of the forthcoming 1987 NMES data tapes and (b) prepare a schedule for the timely release of the National Medical Expenditure Survey data tapes, prepare these public use data tapes as soon as feasible after the reference period, and make them available to the policy and research communities outside the National Center for Health Services Research.

Timely Data from the Medicare Statistical System

The Medicare Statistical System was designed to provide data to measure and evaluate the operation and effectiveness of the Medicare program. It has also been a major source of information for evaluating many policy questions relating to equity and efficiency of the Medicare program. For example, data on the distribution of Medicare reimbursements for survivors and decedents and by type of service provide useful information on the high use of medical care services in the last year of life. Medical reimbursements per capita by state and county are useful measures of equity. Provider certification data related to population are important measures of the supply of facilities and services and their variation across the country. Geographic variations in surgical procedures among the elderly are important indicators of practice patterns.

The statistical system is a by-product of three administrative record systems that are centrally maintained in the operation of the Medicare program: (1) the Health Insurance Master File, which contains a record of each person who is enrolled in Medicare, (2) the Provider of Service File, which contains information on every hospital, skilled nursing facility, home health agency, independent laboratory, and other institutional provider that has been certified to participate in the program, and (3) the Utilization File, which is based on the Medicare billing information. Since each record in the utilization file contains the beneficiary's claim number and the provider's number, the utilization records can be matched to the enrollment and provider records. This then provides the basis for developing population-based statistics or provider-based statistics.

In the past, HCFA has produced a variety of reports, including annual Medicare Program Statistics, Health Care Financing Review, Health Care Financing Notes, Health Care Financing Grants and Contracts Reports series, Medicare Reimbursements by State and County Facilities certified under the Medicare Program, and Enrollees under the program. The latest published data are the Annual Medicare Program Statistics for 1984.

> **Recommendation 8.6:** The panel recommends that the Health Care Financing Administration devote more resources, including budget and staff, to the timely release, publication, and analysis of data from the Medicare Statistical System, including national and geographic data on enrollees, providers, and reimbursements.

Improved Access to Medicare Data

The volume of data potentially available from the MSS is large and especially useful for evaluating different aspects of the Medicare programs as noted above. The panel commends the Health Care Financing Administration for its efforts to develop useful files such as the Medicare Automated Retrieval System and the Medicare Provider Analysis and Review (MEDPAR). The MEDPAR Public Use File is a national sample of bills for short-stay hospital inpatient services for 20 percent of the Medicare beneficiaries selected according to predetermined digits of the health insurance claim number. The elements of the bill (SSA-1453) contained in the file are: age, sex, Medicare status code; length of stay, discharge status; total and Medicare-covered charges; principal diagnosis in ICD-9-CM code and DRG code. The file has been maintained annually since 1980.

Despite the obvious attractiveness of the Medicare files for analytic purposes, it must be noted that these files were established primarily to assist with administration and monitoring of the Medicare program. In order to make the Medicare administrative data more accessible and less costly for research use, a new file has been designed—the Medicare Automated Data Retrieval System. The MADRS is intended to reorganize and merge Medicare Part A and Part B claims files to shorten search time. Beginning with the 1982 data year, this file will contain all Medicare claims data and patient provider identifiers. The claims records in the Medicare files will be sorted first by year of service rendered, next by geographic region of residence of beneficiaries, and then by the health insurance number of the beneficiaries. It will be possible to create a longitudinal file for cohort analysis by combining data in the annual files (Office of Technology Assessment, 1985a, Appendix E:199; Lichtenstein et al., no date; National Research Council, 1986).

The MADRS file will enable researchers to identify groups of special interest and analyze them by age, sex, and/or admitting diagnosis, for example, and examine the care they have received over time. The development of the Medicare Automated Data Retrieval System is a positive step toward facilitating the analysis of Medicare data, thus gaining a better understanding of health services utilization trends among the elderly.

Recommendation 8.7: The panel recommends that the Health Care Financing Administration develop files designed for easy access to the Medicare Statistical System, including the Medicare Automated Data Retrieval System, that would facilitate use by researchers for policy analysis related to the Medicare program.

Making data from administrative records available to researchers would be expected to result in information useful to both program agencies and policy makers. The Health Care Financing Administration should develop new approaches to improving access by nonfederal users, such as interns and postdoctoral fellows. More use should also be made of the Intergovernmental Personnel Act of 1970, which provides for agreements between federal agencies and state agencies for assignment or exchange of personnel for a specified period. Such exchanges are usually beneficial to both agencies.

Recommendation 8.8: The panel recommends that the Health Care Financing Administration complete the development of the Medicare Automated Data Retrieval System and maintain it on a current basis.

The Health Care Financing Administration Data System for Capitation

An alternative to fee-for-service reimbursement types of insurance is payment on a per capita basis without regard to the volume or type of service. HMOs have been the major systems that charge a fixed monthly fee (capitation fee) to cover all services except for small copayments. With the passage of the Tax Equity and Fiscal Responsibility Act (TEFRA) in 1982 and the issuance of regulations to implement the HMO provisions of TEFRA in January 1984, the number of HMOs participating in Medicare is expected to grow, as is the number of Medicare enrollees in HMOs. There are currently over 1 million Medicare beneficiaries in HMOs (i.e., prepayment for services). Historically, the Medicare Statistical System has provided summary data on beneficiary demographics and extensive data on the use and costs of Medicare benefits on both the beneficiary level and on the level of institutional providers (hospitals, skilled nursing facilities, home health agencies, hospital outpatient departments). The data have been used for program administration, monitoring, and evaluation. However, the use and cost data are by and large derived from claims for payment of service. Capitated payment systems such as HMOs are paid an overall capitation amount by HCFA so there is no transaction record to describe services rendered and payment made. As more beneficiaries leave the fee-for-service sector, the information gap on use of services will grow.

Data will be needed from HMOs to monitor the care received by beneficiaries of public programs and to gather information required for setting and evaluating capitation rates. The panel recognizes that, in some cases, HMOs may have to establish new data systems to obtain such information. HCFA will need data from HMOs to address a number of issues, differences in patterns of care by plan type, access to specialty services, and monitoring the appropriateness of payment formulas for HMOs. Some of these issues are common to the fee-for-service sector, but others, such as biased selection, are unique to capitation.

> **Recommendation 8.9:** The panel recommends that the Health Care Financing Administration develop a data system for information on Medicare beneficiaries in capitated systems that is beneficiary-based, able to accommodate different types of capitated plans, reflect differences in services offered and in cost sharing, and utilizes uniform and consistent data definitions and formats among different types of plans.

This recommendation complements the more general Recommendation 9.1 to modify national health data systems to reflect changing patterns and sources of service delivery.

Disability-Medicare Linked File

The long-term effects of disability are an important component of functional limitations in the older population, medical care, utilization, and expenditures. The Social Security Administration, which administers the Disability Insurance program, maintains a Continuous Disability History Sample, a file stratified by state and including from 5 to 20 percent of each state's newly disabled individuals who have been determined to be eligible for future benefits awarded to the disabled population. The disabled are eligible for benefits under the Medicare program two years after the disability insurance award is made. In 1983, Medicare per capita expenditures for the disabled ($1,900) at ages under 65 (excluding persons covered under the End Stage Renal Disease program) were higher than for the elderly ($1,724). The Medicare disabled, as a group, accounted for about $5.5 billion of a total $57.4 billion, for the entire Medicare program (Health Care Financing Administration, 1985a). As the disabled population ages, they will constitute a significant subgroup of the elderly population requiring considerable medical care outlays. The Medicare experience of the disabled population under age 65 should be analyzed as a basis for forecasting their medical care utilization patterns and future Medicare outlays when they become 65 and older.

HCFA has developed a file detailing the Medicare experience for 1977-1981 for the cohort of persons becoming entitled to disability benefits in 1972. Utilization and expenditures for Medicare-covered services can thus be related to the diagnosis or type of disability that justified the disability award. Analyses of the linked file is now under way. When it is completed, it can serve as a baseline for a more current study, using the population entitled to disability benefits in 1980 linked to 1982-1986 data.

> **Recommendation 8.10:** The panel recommends that studies of the Continuous Disability History Sample linked to Medicare files be fully supported jointly by the Health Care Financing Administration and the Social Security Administration and that a public use tape be prepared for this linked file with identifiers deleted as necessary to comply with confidentiality requirements.

Data for Policy Analysis of the Prospective Payment System

In 1983, HCFA introduced the prospective payment system (PPS) for reimbursing hospitals treating Medicare patients. Each discharged patient is classified into one of 468 diagnoses called diagnosis-related groups based on the information on the hospital bill. The hospital is paid the fixed predetermined amount for that DRG.

Implementation of the prospective payment system has resulted in shortening the average length of stay for Medicare patients. Studies are under way to determine whether patients discharged under PPS were not yet ready for self-care and, if so, where they obtained needed care. The HCFA hospital bill includes items for patients discharged to home under care of organized home health services, discharged to skilled nursing home or to intermediate nursing facility, in addition to the items on the Uniform Hospital Discharge Data Set (UHDDS): routine discharge, left against medical advice, discharged to another short-term hospital, discharged to a long-term care institution, died, and not stated.

The original Uniform Hospital Discharge Data Set was promulgated by the secretary of the Department of Health, Education, and Welfare in 1974. The additional detail for "Disposition of Patient" has been made part of the Uniform Bill required for each hospital discharge by HCFA.

The UHDDS was reviewed without change in 1980 (U.S. Department of Health and Human Services, 1980c) and by the Health Information Policy Council in 1984 (Federal Register, July 31, 1985:31038-9). The council review served to clarify some categories and definitions but did not add more detailed categories to "Disposition of Patient." More detailed information, similar to that on the Medicare billing form, could be useful in studying length of hospital stay in conjunction with diagnostic information (including multiple diagnoses) and severity of illness. Diagnostic information is available in hospital bill reports, which provide for up to five diagnoses for each discharge, and in the National Hospital Discharge Survey, which provides for seven. Severity of illness information is not available currently for analysis.

Recommendation 8.11: The panel recommends that the National Committee on Vital and Health Statistics reconsider the Disposition of Patient items on the Uniform Hospital Discharge Data Set with reference to the changing data needs resulting from implementation of the prospective payment system.

Medicaid Data

The Medicaid program is unlike the Medicare program, in which data are available on the individual elderly or disabled and his or her use of medical care services. Medicaid is administered by the states, and HCFA does not receive any person-level data on Medicaid eligibles, recipients, or payments made for their medical services. The lack of detailed and uniform administrative data has limited evaluation of the program at the national level.

The Medicaid Tape-To-Tape Project was initiated to expand HCFA's ability to collect data to analyze the Medicaid program. The main data base consists of 100-percent data from five participating states (California, Georgia, Michigan, New York, and Tennessee) in uniform codes and formats. These states cover about one-third of the national Medicaid population. States send HCFA their Medicaid Management Information System (MMIS) tapes, which are edited into a comparable format for analysis. Uniform files are produced for each participating state and year. Separated files are maintained for enrollment, claims, and provider data. Claims, provider, and reimbursements can be linked to the Medicaid enrollee who received the service and to the provider who furnished it. The 1980-1982 data from the five participating states have been collected and uniform files completed; 1983-1984 data from participating states are being collected at this time.

The tapes prepared by HCFA contain utilization and expenditure information on all Medicaid enrollees in the five participating states. The tapes include four different person identifiers on each enrollee, making it possible to link the data with other data sets and national surveys. Experimental studies conducted inside and outside the Health Care Financing Administration—some of which have involved elderly utilization patterns—have yielded high match rates. In addition, for that portion of elderly Medicaid users who are also enrolled in Medicare in these five states (a subset of the "dually eligible" elderly), it has also been found that their Medicaid and Medicare records can be reliably linked, with match rates as high as the high 70s to the low 90s (personal communication, David Baugh, Health Care Financing Administration). HCFA staff are currently working on linking the Medicaid tape-to-tape records to the Medicare files.

Recommendation 8.12: The panel recommends that the Medicaid Tape-to-Tape Project be continued, and that the Health Care Financing Administration continue to conduct studies on utilization patterns and expenditures of the elderly using this data base and create sample files and public use tapes for use by outside researchers.

HCFA has undertaken a project to modernize the agency's information system called Project to Redesign Information System Management (PRISM) (Health Care Financing Administration, 1985b). The first stage, development of the system's design concept, was completed in April 1985. Implementation of the entire system is projected for installation by the end of fiscal 1989. Among its goals are increased support of the Medicare/Medicaid Statistical Systems. Completion of PRISM will facilitate implementation of the panel's recommendation.

Medicaid Eligibility Quality Control System

The Medicaid Eligibility Quality Control system (MEQC) was designed to ensure that public funds are spent only on behalf of people who are eligible under federal and state law. It is concerned with identifying ineligible people enrolled in Medicaid and with payments made in error to providers on behalf of those persons. State-level samples are drawn monthly from the Medicaid population in both civilian and institutionalized settings, using the Medicaid case as the sampling unit. The sample cases are checked for errors.

In 1982, the federal agencies responsible for the AFDC, Medicaid, and Food Stamps programs completed a seven-year effort to design a single form: the Integrated Quality Control System (IQCS) form for use in all programs. Although the medical claims may not be useful because they are added together for the entire case and are not collected on a person-by-person basis, there are other valuable data on the form, such as demographics, detailed income and assets, employment, occupation, spend-down amounts, insurance coverage, utilization, diagnoses, and types of services. The IQCS forms are used extensively by the research units in the AFDC and Food Stamps programs, but HCFA does not use them for research.

The panel recognizes that the MEQC system may have potential for research purposes. A national data base on Medicaid cases could be constructed from the re-review sample (a subsample of the IQC sample), which might be less costly than other alternatives, such as sample surveys of individuals and their associated claims or obtaining the entire claims files. Many issues need to be resolved, and despite its interesting prospects, the panel is not making a recommendation on the MEQC system. The National Research Council's Panel on Quality Control of Family Assistance Programs recently completed a study of other aspects of monitoring and analytic needs of the MEQC system (Kramer, 1988).

Data Resources Required to Study the Medicaid Spend-down Phenomenon

A small group of the elderly have medical expenses that exceed the coverage provided by Medicare and any private insurance they may have. These expenses are chiefly incurred for nursing home services. The costs are high, may continue for years, and are rarely covered by private insurance. Although many elderly people think nursing home services are covered by Medicare, they are not. The Medicaid program is the principal source of public financing for nursing home care, paying for services provided to the indigent and the "medically needy"—those whose income and assets fall below a legally defined level.

Many elderly persons deplete both income and assets in meeting their medical expenses. When they have reached the "medically needy" level, they become eligible for the Medicaid program in the District of Columbia and in the 30 states that have programs for the medically needy. Medicaid then covers all their medical expenses, with few exceptions. Income from pensions or Social Security benefits paid to retired wage-earners who need nursing home care may support not only the retired person but also the spouse and other dependents. When the source of support for a family must spend-down to required levels for nursing home care, the family may be left with insufficient income for survival. To revise the legislation for eligibility for Medicaid to eliminate family hardship, data will be required on how often spend-down occurs, the amount of out-of-pocket expenses paid before the Medicaid program takes over, and the effect of the spend-down on other family members.

There are two sources of data for persons in nursing homes. One is the National Nursing Home Survey. In 1985, this survey included an admissions component that collected data for a sample of admissions and was designed to produce estimates on the spend-down issue.

A second source of data is the Medicaid Quality Control sample. The sample collects information (among other items) on how eligibility was established for Medicaid. Information on persons involved in the spend-down can be compiled for the 5 percent of Medicaid beneficiaries who are in nursing homes and are selected in the Quality Control sample of 400,000 persons nationwide.

Information about the effect of spend-down on the family may be obtained from two ongoing surveys. The Survey of Income and Program Participation in its health care module collects information on insurance coverage, including Medicare and Medicaid for the sample household. It should be possible to examine the detailed data on income and assets in relation to health insurance coverage during the 2 1/2 year period in which the same panel remains in the sample. Changes in coverage and assets could be related. The value of this data source would be greatly enhanced if the recommendation in Chapter 10 to increase the size of the sample of persons of age 65 and over is implemented. Sample augmentation would double the number of those ages 75-84, and 85 and over—the ages in which nursing home admissions are highest.

The NHIS Supplement on Aging, and the subsequent follow-up through the Longitudinal Study on Aging, will also develop information on the family and the individual admitted to the nursing home, if panel recommendation 7.3 on a biennial follow-up is implemented.

The panel reaffirms the need for the expansion of the SIPP sample of the elderly, and for continuation of the Longitudinal Study on Aging in order to study the spend-down phenomenon. In addition, data from the Medicaid quality control data base and from the Nursing Home Survey should be analyzed for information on this problem.

Private Insurance Data

Although at least 25 companies now offer free-standing long-term care insurance, insurers are reluctant to offer and market long-term care policies aggressively. Insurance industry representatives point to concerns about adverse selection, insurance-induced demand, pricing difficulties, and lack of consumer education as barriers to product development. Some insurers have expressed fear that the open-ended liability that can result from long-term care policies could be financially devastating to their companies. There is also concern about the long lag time between purchase of policies and payment of substantial long-term costs and that nonmedical, personal services such as homemaker care and respite care are not insurable.

Insurers also find that actuarial estimates and premium determinations for long-term care policies are difficult to make. Minimal data are available on costs and utilization of long-term care insurance, and very little of the data reflects actual experience. Some are concerned that problems could occur if only high-risk individuals are attracted to long-term care insurance. At present, there is no reliable actuarial model applicable to a long-term care policy that would differentiate the high-risk purchaser from the low-risk one and allow for a variable rate scale.

Private insurance companies are beginning to gain experience with long-term care insurance. The panel recognizes the need for improved data on utilization of covered services, costs, risk management, marketing, and the impact of long-term care coverage.

Cost-of-Illness Data

Cost-of-illness data play an important role in decision making regarding the allocation of resources in the health sector. Illnesses, such as Alzheimer's disease, that primarily affect the elderly will require more resources in the future with the growing number of elderly persons who may be at risk. Alzheimer's disease, affecting an estimated 1.5 million Americans, has become a major priority for federal research organizations (e.g., the National Institute on Aging, the National Institute of Neurological and Communicative Disorders and Stroke, and the National Institute of Mental Health). Many other diseases and impairments that affect the elderly include heart disease, cancer, arthritis, stroke, as well as visual and hearing impairments.

In addition to data on prevalence, incidence, and use of medical care and long-term care services for the elderly suffering from these and other conditions, the costs of these conditions are needed by policy makers, health planners, and researchers to set priorities, make program policy decisions, and prepare and deliver congressional testimony to support program policy decisions and agency budgets.

The economic costs of illness represent the monetary burden on society of illness and premature death. They represent foregone alternatives and are measured in terms of the direct and indirect costs. Direct costs are the value of resources that could be allocated to other uses in the absence of disease, and indirect costs are the value of lost output because of cessation or reduction of productivity due to morbidity and mortality. Morbidity costs are lost wages for people unable to work due to illness and disability and an imputed value for those persons too sick to perform their usual housekeeping services. Mortality costs are the present value of future earnings lost for people who die prematurely, employing discounting to convert a stream of future earnings into present values.

Total economic costs of illness in 1980 amounted to $455 billion based on a 4 percent discount rate of the value of productivity foregone in succeeding years as a result of premature mortality in that year. The elderly (persons age 65 and over) comprised 11.3 percent of the total population in 1980 and 18.2 percent of the total economic costs (Rice et al., 1985).

The rankings by major diagnostic category of the economic costs of illness vary substantially by age. For the population under age 65, the medical condition that ranks highest in economic costs is "injury and poisoning," costing $78 billion, accounting for 21 percent of the total for this age group, and reflecting the relatively high value of lost productivity for the large number of premature deaths at younger ages from this cause. Diseases of the circulatory system rank second in economic costs for persons under age 65, representing 15 percent of the total. For the elderly, the economic costs of diseases of circulatory system far outrank all other diseases, amounting to $29 billion, or 35 percent of the total. In second place are neoplasms, constituting 11 percent of total economic costs for the elderly.

These cost-of-illness estimates are for the major diagnostic categories and are not disaggregated to specific diseases. There have been more than 200 separate cost-of-illness studies in the last 20 years (Hu and Sandifer, 1981). Some of these are national in scope, but most are limited to a selected population or geographic area, and all but a few are restricted to one or a few disease categories. Varying methodologies are used so that the costs of different diseases cannot be compared.

Estimation of the costs of illness depend to a great extent on the data available and on the methodologies used. Although the U.S. Public Health Service has developed guidelines for estimation of the costs of illness (Hodgson and Meiners, 1982), few studies follow them rigorously. For the further development of cost-of-illness studies, data will be available from several surveys including the 1987 National Medical Care Expenditure Survey, the 1985 National Nursing Home Survey, the annual National Hospital Discharge Survey, and the annual National Health Interview Survey. Additional sources of data are the Medicare, Medicaid, and other public program administrative records.

Recommendation 8.13: The panel recommends that the National Center for Health Services Research, the National Center for Health Statistics, and the Health Care Financing Administration continue to collect the detailed data necessary to estimate the economic costs of illnesses, especially those affecting the elderly population, and that the National Center for Health Services Research support cost-of-illness studies using available guidelines for uniform methodology.

9
Health Services Utilization

INTRODUCTION

The amount and types of health care services used by older adults is influenced by many factors. Although the need for health services and the frequency and intensity of service utilization are clearly related to health status and level of impairment or disability, many factors unrelated to health needs per se also play important roles. Among these are public policies that specify the types of services and providers covered by public funds, cost-sharing provisions, the supply of alternative sources and types of care; living arrangements and access to informal care; the availability of adequate numbers of trained personnel; advances or changes in health care technology and delivery systems; and the attitudes and values of potential recipients and providers of care.

The issues involved are shaped largely by public policies dealt with previously in the discussions of long-term care in Chapter 7 and the financing of health care services for the elderly in Chapter 8. The questions that follow recast many of those raised earlier to sharpen consideration of requirements for policy-relevant data on health services for the elderly generally, i.e., those who receive episodic care as well as those who are in need of long-term care. Major policy issues that need to be addressed through special research and demonstration programs are listed first and these are followed by questions that are clearly related and should be answerable through information systems.

- How do benefit provisions and cost sharing under Medicare, including the deductibles, affect the rates of use of different types of health services and providers?
- What gaps in Medicare are being filled by supplemental private health insurance; how widespread is this type of coverage; and what effect does such coverage have on the utilization of health services?
- How does the supply of alternative sources and types of care influence the use of health services; what sectors of health care are most affected now; how will trends toward increased home care, adult day care programs, and other alternative types of services alter levels and patterns of utilization of health services?
- How are the content, type, and place of care affected by the use of physicians and allied health personnel trained in gerontology? How will future requirements for health care resources be affected by the increased availability of such personnel now being projected?
- To what extent are advances in diagnostic and therapeutic health care technology reaching the elderly; how are they affecting utilization of health services subsequent to treatment; what is the role of government in determining appropriate access of the elderly to health care technology established as cost-effective?
- How are changes in the structure of health care systems and reimbursement arrangements, e.g., capitation payments to HMOs and preferred provider organizations influencing the patterns of health care utilization; how effective are these changes in meeting health care needs of the elderly?oWhat is the effect of changes in benefits, cost sharing, and other cost-containment measures, such as prospective payment systems (e.g., diagnosis-related group in the hospital), on rates and sources of care used, and how rapidly do these changes occur?

Need for Services

Need can be viewed from two vantage points, that of the provider and that of the consumer. In the former instance, what is often meant by need is the health care expert's view of requirements for primary or secondary prevention of disease, diagnosis, treatment, or rehabilitation in the presence of specified signs, symptoms, or conditions. Recourse to health services is expected to result in some benefit to the patient, the degree of certainty of benefit varying with knowledge of natural history of the condition and the availability of interventions that are effective at different stages of the condition. Furthermore, agreement may be greater on whether care should be obtained than on the nature, source, or volume of care required (or its outcome). Nevertheless, standards exist for certain types of services, as reflected by the prospective payment system for hospital care as well as for treatment of specific conditions such as hypertension and other chronic conditions.

From the consumer's standpoint, the concern is with a complex set of perceptions, values, and other factors that facilitate or create barriers to health services. The end point is the observed utilization of services and care identified by the consumer as needed but not obtained. This is independent of the provider's appraisal of the appropriateness of the care sought.

Of interest is the repeated observation that older persons on average tend to view their health positively, although less often, than younger persons. Responses to the 1982 National Health Interview Survey indicate that some 65 percent of elderly persons living in the community viewed their health as good to excellent when compared to others of their own age; and only 35 percent reported their health as fair or poor (U.S. Congress, Senate, 1986a). This information is subject to a variety of interpretations, but self-assessed or perceived health status is associated with the use of health care services as measured, for instance, by rates of physician utilization (Crozier, 1985; Waldo and Lazenby, 1984).

Clearly, the extent to which the elderly use the formal health care system, including noninstitutional and short- and long-term institutional care, is related to the level and complexity of their medical needs, which, on average, increase with age. Those with manifest disability tend to make the most intensive use of health care service (Lubitz and Prihoda, 1984). Utilization rates tend to be highest during the last year or two of life (Lubitz and Prihoda, 1984; Gornick et al., 1985), and for some types of services, e.g., hospital and nursing home care, they are far greater among the oldest-old than among those ages 65-74 (U.S. Congress, Senate, 1986a; National Center for Health Statistics, 1981).

Impact of Public Policies

There is no question that increased access to care afforded the elderly by the Medicare and Medicaid programs enacted in 1965 has had a large impact on the use of health care services by the elderly, both as regards the types of services consumed and the frequency and intensity of service utilization. Rates of hospital and nursing home use by the elderly, for example, increased substantially between the late 1960s and the late 1970s (Rice and Feldman, 1983; Gornick et al., 1985). Much of the increase in service utilization of hospitals, skilled and intermediate care nursing facilities, home health care, and physicians' services, for instance, has been attributed to previously unmet needs (Rabin, 1985). Changes in coverage provisions and reimbursement rates, for both the federal Medicare program and the federal-state Medicaid program, are likely to affect future utilization patterns, as well as the providers of care, as they have in the past (see Chapter 8). The Medicaid program already varies considerably among states since the states have significant flexibility in determining eligibility for assistance, the scope of benefits provided, and reimbursement rates for these services. This verification may well increase as states attempt to curtail costs with differential effects on access to medical care on the part of the poor, including the poor elderly. Medicare coverage for services provided to the elderly by HMOs and other capitated plans can be expected to affect the types of services consumed by the elderly as well as their mode of provision. The federally initiated DRG system for reimbursing hospitals for the care they provide to the elderly under Medicare, as well as the federally encouraged increasing use of prospective payment systems for health care generally, are other major policy changes that affect the demand and supply of services available to the elderly. (For an analysis of the potential impact of hospital DRGs on access to inpatient hospital and other types of care by the elderly and vulnerable elderly groups such as the frail, disabled, alcoholic, poor, and mentally ill, see Office of Technology Assessment, 1985a).

Federal policies affect both the supply and training of geriatric manpower, which has implications for service availability and utilization. At the state level, certificate of need (CON) requirements for authorization to build or expand hospitals and nursing homes can greatly constrict or enhance the supply of services available to meet the needs of the elderly, and thus affect service utilization. The supply of nursing home beds available to impaired elderly and other disabled persons is determined in part by state CON policies (Feder and Scanlon, 1980).

Supply of Alternative Sources and Types of Care

The availability of substitute, or alternative types of health care services or facilities for persons with particular health needs or limitations in function affects the utilization of these services and facilities in complex and incompletely understood ways. The chronic care needs of the moderately impaired elderly—assistance with activities of daily living or instrumental activities of daily living, for example— in contrast to their strictly medical care needs, can be met in a variety of settings. These settings include intermediate care nursing facilities, retirement communities, adult day care centers or programs, or the home with the assistance of family members or with community-provided services such as meals-on-wheels and visiting nurses. The extent to which each or any of these types of services or support systems will be used by an individual or group of persons similarly disabled depends in part on their availability within the community, in part on the ease of access to these and other kinds of arrangements, and in part on the financing mechanisms.

Care for the acutely ill as well may be provided in more than one setting or type of facility—in a hospital as an inpatient (as is typical), in a hospital as an outpatient, in a skilled nursing facility, in a physician's office, or in the home—depending on the availability of these different sources of care, the wishes of the individual and family, and financial factors and insurance coverage.

Living Arrangements and Access to Informal Care

Living arrangements and access to informal care provided by relatives or friends also affect the demand for formal health care and health-related services. A recent study found that elderly people living alone were at greater risk of institutionalization than comparably disabled people of the same age living with one or more other persons after controlling for variables such as age, medical status, and functional status (Branch and Jette, 1982). For example, elderly persons who are married and/or live with or near adult relatives— particularly their adult children—are less likely to be consumers of formal health services than those who live alone. "At any level of need, the probability of formal service is lowest for those elderly who live with either spouses or other relatives" (Soldo and Manton, 1985:306). The family clearly plays an important role as determiner of service needs, finders of services, and brokers for its elderly relatives.

Demographic trends will influence the availability of informal sources of care for the elderly. Future cohorts of U.S. elderly persons will be larger than the present cohort, and the greatest increase in size and percentage of the entire U.S. population will occur among the oldest old. As the population ages, successive cohorts of potential informal caregivers, such as spouses or adult children of ill or impaired elderly people, will be older as well and possibly less able to care for their elderly relatives because of their own health limitations. In addition, families are having fewer children and, as discussed in Chapter 2, the number of elderly women living alone is increasing rapidly.

Availability of Trained Personnel

Utilization of health services by the elderly who have particular combinations of medical problems is affected by the availability of health and medical care personnel who are trained to meet the health care needs unique to the elderly population. Increasingly, questions are being raised about the quality of care provided to the elderly by both primary care providers and specialists, in both institutional and noninstitutional settings (Kane et al., 1980; Institute of Medicine, 1986). Moreover, the diagnosis and management of diseases and illnesses common among older adults, such as Alzheimer's disease, require special training in geriatrics. While information on current numbers of appropriately trained personnel is limited (National Institute on Aging, 1984b), most sources concur that inadequate attention has been paid to ensuring an adequate supply of trained practitioners, including generalists, specialists, and academics, to provide care to the elderly and to advance the knowledge base (see, for example, National Institute on Aging, 1984b; National Institute on Aging, 1985; Minaker and Rowe, 1985). Projected increases in the elderly population, particularly among those age 75 and over, reinforce the need to attend to the personnel and training issue.

Technological Advances or Changes

Utilization of health services by the elderly is also affected by the introduction, availability, and diffusion of new medical technologies, including techniques, drugs, equipment, and procedures used by health care personnel in prevention, diagnosis and screening, treatment, or rehabilitation (see Young, 1985). The development and availability of CT (computed tomography) scanning and NMR (nuclear magnetic resonance) for the detection of tumors, cardiac pacemaker implant surgery, coronary artery bypass surgery to relieve angina pectoris, and hip arthroplasty (total hip replacement) are examples of technological innovations and procedures that have grown rapidly in recent years. Cataract surgery with lens implant, coronary artery bypass surgery, and hip arthroplasty are surgical procedures that were relatively new in 1972 but whose use increased rapidly for people age 65 and over between 1972 and 1981. For example, from 1972 to 1981, hip arthroplasties increased in number by 244 percent for people age 65 and over, and 509 percent for those age 74 and over. And by 1981, an estimated 250,000 people age 65 and over had a lens implant—a rare procedure in 1972 (Valvona and Sloan, 1985).

Attitudes and Values of Potential Recipients and Providers of Care

Attitudes regarding formal caregivers and the perceived value of formal health care services by older adults affect health care utilization rates. Of major importance are perceptions and attitudes concerning the nature of an "illness," which may be very different from the medically defined "disease" diagnosed within the health care setting. For example, the consumption of mental health services by the noninstitutionalized elderly is lower than the prevalence of mental illness or psychiatric disorder would warrant (Shapiro, 1986; Hall, 1983; Taeuber, 1983). The presence of unmet need for mental health services among the elderly may also, or alternatively, signal "a lack of recognition or willingness to accept the presence of a mental or emotional problem that should be brought to medical attention and the infrequency of detection of an emotional problem by the primary care clinician" (Shapiro, 1986). Even when the elderly seek care, health care professionals often prefer to spend time with younger patients whose ailments are more likely to be curable than with elderly patients needing chronic care (Kane et al., 1981; Office of Technology Assessment, 1985b). It should also be recognized that Medicare coverage of mental health problems is much more limited than coverage under many general health insurance programs.

DATA SOURCES ON HEALTH CARE UTILIZATION

The remainder of this chapter reviews the adequacy of federal data sources on the use of available health care services by the elderly, both through the formal and the informal health care systems. The discussion is organized around four major issues: the availability of trained health personnel to work with the elderly; effects of changes in the organization, provision, and coverage of health care services; the relationship between health status and health service utilization; and equity in access to care.

Information on health services utilization by the elderly is generated by three types of federal data collection activities: provider-based surveys, general population surveys, and administrative records maintained by federal agencies. Provider-based surveys generate information about health services utilization by surveying samples of providers of care, such as hospitals, physicians, and nursing homes. Population-based surveys obtain such information by interviewing or making observations on samples of individuals selected from the general population or certain segments of it. These two approaches to data collection are complementary and, in fact, some surveys sample both providers and populations—that is, they have both provider and population components as integral parts of the survey. Administrative records are tools developed by federal agencies mainly for the purpose of managing and monitoring federal programs, e.g., records maintained by the Health Care Financing Administration to manage and monitor the Medicare program. These records are an important source of data on the use of health services by the elderly.

Data Related to Health Personnel Trained to Work With the Elderly

The quality of care and the quality of life for the elderly with multiple and complex medical problems are enhanced when medical care is provided by health care professionals, and allied personnel who are trained and experienced in geriatrics and gerontology (Kane et al., 1980). Both professionals, such as physicians and social workers, and support personnel, including nurses' aides and home health workers who provide hands-on and continuing care, play a large role in the everyday life of older persons who are frail or ill.

Comprehensive data on the numbers of professionals and allied health personnel who presently render direct care to the elderly do not exist. Nor is there information on the numbers that will be needed in the future to meet the health needs of the rapidly growing elderly sector of the population. Some federal agencies, such as the Bureau of Health Professions of the Health Resources and Services Administration (U.S. Public Health Service), have attempted to collect some data. In 1983 and 1984, the Bureau sampled licensed practical nurses (LPNs) and registered nurses to determine how many work in settings that render care to the elderly (personal communication, Thomas Hatch, Chief, Bureau of Health Professions). Data sets, privately generated for internal use by professional societies or associations, generally do not identify members who work with or provide services to the elderly. An exception is the American Medical Association's survey of its member physicians, which collects data on the numbers who report a primary interest in geriatrics (National Institute on Aging, 1984b). Moreover, many private data sources have typically not been developed as information bases for public use.

The Health Research Extension Act of 1985 (U.S. Congress, 1985), Section 8, called for a Study of Personnel for Health Needs of the Elderly. It directed the secretary of the U.S. Department of Health and Human Services to "conduct a study on the adequacy and availability of personnel to meet the current and projected health needs (including needs for home and community-based care) of elderly Americans through the year 2020" (U.S. Congress, 1985). Chapter 5 includes a brief description of the contents of the secretary's report.

The study defines health personnel broadly to include not only the usual professionals who deal with and render care to the elderly in both institutional and noninstitutional settings (e.g., physicians, registered nurses, social workers), but also nursing home and hospital administrators, specialized geriatricians, all varieties of acute and long-term care nurse and allied personnel below the bachelor's level (such as LPNs and aides), and health researchers, among others.

Other noteworthy activities include the voluntary efforts of those professional associations and membership organizations that currently collect, or attempt to collect, information on the health and related services their members provide to the elderly and the settings in which they render such services. The panel encourages these associations and organizations to continue and refine their data collection activities in this area and suggests that others join them in collecting such information on their own members.

The panel is concerned, however, about the lack of routine and standardized data collection efforts by the federal government needed to determine the current and future estimated supply of professionals and support personnel who are engaged in providing health care to the elderly. The panel encourages federal agencies to give further attention to mechanisms by which such information can be generated.

Measuring the Effects of Changes in the Organization, Provision, and Coverage of Health Care Services

Changes in Provider Characteristics

Changes in the organization and provision of health care and related services, as discussed more fully in Chapter 5, are having and will continue to have a considerable impact on the service utilization patterns not only of the general population but also of the elderly. Provision must be made to monitor their impact over time through various continuing and periodic surveys, both provider- and population-based.

> **Recommendation 9.1:** The panel recommends that federal agencies give high priority to reviewing and modifying the contents of administrative record systems, provider-based surveys, and, to the extent feasible, population-based surveys to reflect the rapidly changing patterns in health service delivery. These modifications should enable respondents and surveyors to distinguish among the various types of health plans in use, including the varieties of capitated plans, and to detect differences in their cost-sharing provisions. Standard definitions and formats for recording the health plan information should be used by all agencies collecting such data.

Physicians and Utilization of Their Services An important source of utilization data is the National Ambulatory Care Survey, which collects data on office visits made by ambulatory patients to nonfederal physicians engaged principally in office-based patient care practice. The unit of analysis for this survey is the physician-patient encounter (National Center for Health Statistics, 1984b).

At present, this survey has several limitations that affect its utility as a major source of national data on the content and volume of physician services received by the elderly and the general population.

One is its periodicity. Instead of being an annual survey with continuous collection of data as initially planned and conducted, it was changed to a triennial survey because of budget considerations in the National Center for Health Statistics (Shapiro, 1984). A second limitation concerns its coverage. At present, the sampling frame for this survey is office-based physicians in solo or group practice (including HMOs). Excluded are physicians whose practice is hospital-based and those who are federally employed. The latter results in a gap in information about service utilization by veterans and dependents of those in military service. The former exclusion means that physician visits of minority populations residing in urban areas are underrepresented because members of such populations are relatively high users of hospital-based physician services, including emergency services. The sampling frame also excludes physician practices in other care settings such as the rapidly expanding surgi-centers, where many procedures formerly performed on an inpatient basis are now taking place. Until surgi-centers are included in NAMCS, it will remain unclear to what extent and for what procedures the elderly are receiving care in these facilities.

A third limitation of this survey as a source of national utilization data on the elderly is that the report form concerning physician visits does not address specific health care needs of the elderly. The inclusion of items, such as whether tests for preventable illnesses and disabilities were performed during the visit, would enhance the utility of this survey for physician-patient encounters that involve older persons (see Chapter 5 for the panel's recommendation pertaining to this aspect of the National Ambulatory Medical Care Survey).

> **Recommendation 9.2:** The panel recommends that the National Ambulatory Medical Care Survey sampling frame be expanded to include physicians practicing in federal hospitals, hospital outpatient clinics, surgi-centers, and other alternative care centers.

Hospitals and Utilization of Their Services The National Hospital Discharge Survey, a continuous survey conducted by the National Center for Health Statistics since 1965, is the primary survey-based source of information on inpatient utilization of short-stay nonfederal hospitals. Its purpose is to produce statistics that are representative of the experience of the U.S. civilian population discharged from short-stay hospitals exclusive of military and Veterans Administration hospitals. It samples discharge record abstracts in a sample of hospitals of various sizes and types of ownership and provides information on the characteristics of patients, their length of stay, diagnoses (including DRGs), surgical procedures, and use of care for the four major geographic regions of the country. In 1984 an estimated 37.2 million patients, including 11.2 million persons age 65 and over, were discharged from such hospitals (National Center for Health Statistics, 1985b).

The sampling frame for the National Hospital Discharge Survey does not include federal providers—a significant gap in view of the demographics of aging veterans. The Veterans Administration, however, does collect information from all its hospitals on a routine basis and for 100 percent of its discharges. The two data collection efforts, while complementary in coverage, have not been coordinated in terms of content and definitions. The panel strongly suggests that the National Center for Health Statistics and the Veterans Administration coordinate their data collection efforts in this area to provide a more comprehensive national picture of hospital utilization by the general population, including the elderly.

National Health Care Survey The National Center for Health Statistics plans to develop an integrated National Health Care Survey by merging over time its four provider-based surveys: the National Hospital Discharge Survey, the National Nursing Home Survey (described in Chapter 7), the National Ambulatory Medical Care Survey (described earlier in this chapter) and the National Master Facility Inventory. These four data systems rely on information from providers of health care, rather than from recipients. The new design will alleviate problems associated with the periodic nature of the current surveys. It would also facilitate expansion of coverage to include sources of care not well addressed currently, for example, HMOs, preferred provider organizations, and additional types of long-term care providers, including home health care agencies, community health centers, and hospices.

According to the fiscal year 1988 issue paper, "Planning for a National Health Care Survey" prepared by National Center for Health Statistics (3/19/86): The National Health Care Survey (NCHS) would be designed to produce annual data on the use of health care and the outcomes of care for all major sectors of the health delivery system. The survey would have two parts:

- Provider Component: Data would be collected from providers about the patient, care provider, financing, and provider characteristics. This component would produce national data on the structure and output of the major sectors of the health care delivery system—hospital care, ambulatory care, and long-term care.

• Patient Follow-On Component: Data would be collected periodically from the patient (possibly by telephone) to determine the long-range outcomes of care and subsequent use of care. This component would produce longitudinal data on quality of care, episodes of care, and the dynamics of the use of health care and its financing. The patient follow-on component could be focused on various dimensions: e.g., provider financing mechanisms, a diagnosis or procedure; a particular demographic group (e.g., aged, poor, minority); discharge to long-term institutional care. The dimensions could be changed periodically to address emerging issues and special topics. Finally, the National Death Index would be searched for mortality status and cause of death information obtained from state health departments.

The integrated sample design, which requires further research, would sample certain geographic areas, and then sample health care providers within the area. The four provider-based surveys would be phased into the integrated survey beginning in fiscal 1988. The design would focus initially on the hospital, next on modification of the NAMCS beginning in 1989, the long-term care elements in 1991, and the NMFI in time to provide a frame for the 1991 long-term care survey. (The panel's Recommendation 7.4 for a three-year cycle for the National Nursing Home Survey is somewhat at variance with this plan.)

The concept underlying the National Health Care Survey is important and holds promise for a significant improvement in information when the initiating observation is a provider-based report of services. Provision is being made for linking the NHCS geographically with the NHIS by using the same area samples for the two surveys. Many methodological issues still need to be resolved and caution should be exercised that the samples are adequate to develop data on age subgroups among the elderly.

Utilization of Dental Care and Services   With the exception of the National Health and Nutrition Examination Survey (discussed below), routine federal data collection efforts in the area of dental health and dental service utilization are meager. While the National Health

Interview Survey (NHIS, see Chapter 3) and the National Ambulatory Medical Care Survey both collect some data about dental visits, and the planned National Medical Expenditure Survey (discussed below) is expected to do so as well, none of them does so in depth. The NHIS did include a supplement on edentulousness in 1971. The National Nursing Home Survey (see Chapter 7), which is designed to be used with the elderly, likewise does not deal with this issue except in a very cursory manner. The Medicare statistical system does not collect such data, because ordinary dental care is not reimbursed under Medicare.

The National Health and Nutrition Examination Survey (described in Chapter 3) is an exception, as far as dental health data are concerned. This survey measures and monitors the health and nutritional status of the U.S. population through direct physical examinations, physiological and biochemical measurements, and personal interviews administered to a sample of the noninstitutionalized population ages 6 months to 74 years. NHANES I (1971-1975) included a dental examination for a part of the sample, and interview items pertaining to perceived dental status and needs on its Health Care Needs Questionnaire (National Center for Health Statistics, 1985c). NHANES II (1976-1980) did not include dental health in its protocols. The Hispanic Health and Nutrition Examination Survey (HHANES), administered from 1982 to 1984 to a sample of Hispanics, included both a dental examination and interview items pertaining not only to perception of dental health, but also to utilization of dental services and barriers to dental care. NHANES III, to begin in 1988, is expected to extend the age of the elderly covered in the sample to 84 (see Chapter 3 for a recommendation concerning sampling of the elderly for NHANES III) and to have a longitudinal component. It will also include a dental examination to determine trends in the prevalence of dental caries and periodontal disease and interview items on dental status very much like those included in NHANES I (personal communication, Kurt Maurer, National Center for Health Statistics). The panel concurs with the National Institute of Dental Research's position regarding the desirability for better national data on the oral health status and dental utilization behaviors of the elderly (U.S. Department of Health and Human Services, 1986b). The need for more extensive inquiry is exceedingly important because dental status and care when needed are central to the ability to digest and gain nutritive value from food, and they affect the quality of life experienced by the elderly.

Recommendation 9.3: The panel recommends that the National Center for Health Statistics develop a set of interview items on dental care utilization of increased relevance to the elderly to be included in the National Health and Nutrition Examination Survey in order to provide more detailed information on dental status and care.

Rehabilitative Care and Services Rehabilitative care and services are provided to persons impaired from acute or chronic disease to help maintain existing residual function, improve function, or restore independent functioning. Such care and services are not intended to cure disease (Office of Technology Assessment, 1985b). They may be heavily technology-intensive or involve the use of very simple devices or none at all. Typically such services are provided by physiatrists (physicians specializing in rehabilitation), physical and occupational therapists, nurses, and speech therapists. Most such services are rendered in hospitals and nursing homes, but they are also provided in the home and at community or senior centers (Office of Technology Assessment, 1985b). Federal data collection efforts are relatively weak in the area of rehabilitative care and services provided to the elderly. Both the National Nursing Home Survey and the Medicare statistical system collect some data—the former in the course of sampling nursing home facilities and the services they provide to individuals, and the latter because Medicare reimburses for some rehabilitative services. Because rehabilitative care and services are so central to the well-being of the disabled and ill elderly—even very small improvements in functioning can make a difference in the quality of life experienced by a nursing home resident—the panel believes that utilization of such services by the elderly should be documented.

Recommendation 9.4: The panel recommends that increased attention be given to the inclusion of questions concerning rehabilitative care in both ongoing provider- and population-based surveys and those that may be initiated in the future.

Rehabilitative care is provided in short- and long-term care facilities as well as on an outpatient basis. Facilities other than nursing homes that provide rehabilitative care as their primary focus are not currently included in the National Master Facility Inventory, which serves as the sampling frame for the National Nursing Home Survey. In Chapter 7 the panel recommended that the inventory be expanded to include many different kinds of facilities that provide long-term care, including those that provide rehabilitative care, to facilitate data collection on elderly residents. Adoption of that recommendation would increase the feasibility of collecting survey data on the utilization of institution-based rehabilitative services by the elderly. Such data would complement the Medicare data that are also available on elderly users of Medicare-reimbursed rehabilitative services.

Utilization of Mental Health Services The extent to which the general population and the elderly use mental health services provided by specialists or general practitioners is not well documented in population- and provider-based surveys such as those conducted by the National Center for Health Statistics. A notable exception is the Epidemiological Catchment Area Program of the National Institute of Mental Health, conducted by academically based investigators in five local areas, in collaboration with the NIMH, as described in Chapter 1. With respect to utilization of services, results show that the elderly are more likely to have unmet need for mental health care than younger persons (Shapiro et al., 1985). They are also far more likely to turn to providers of general medical services than mental health specialists when they seek care for a mental or emotional problem (Shapiro, 1984).

Important as the ECA is, there remains a need for periodic information on a national scale concerning the extent to which the elderly and the population generally receive mental health services and from which sectors of care.

> **Recommendation 9.5:** The panel recommends that the National Center for Health Statistics explore with the National Institute of Mental Health means by which the use of mental health services by older adults, whether provided by specialty or general health care practitioners, can be disaggregated from their use of other health services in national surveys, both population- and provider-based.

Changes in Utilization Patterns

The dynamic nature of financing and delivery of health care discussed in previous chapters may be expected to have both short-term and long-term effects on patterns of utilization of a broad spectrum of ambulatory and institutional care. The longitudinal and cross-sectional periodic surveys already considered are designed to meet the need for this type of information.

It should be noted that while the National Medical Expenditure Survey described in Chapter 8 is directed primarily at economic issues, it is designed to provide extensive health services utilization data on many components and sources of care relevant to the elderly. Current plans focus on information for two age groups, 65-74 and 75 and over. However, since the age group 85 and over is the most rapidly growing segment of the population and the group that makes the greatest use of health care services, it will be critically important in future surveys to collect information on the use of health care services by this age group. Therefore, the panel reiterates its recommendation for augmentation of the sample of the aged population in future national medical expenditure surveys (Recommendation 8.2). A potentially useful approach for obtaining a larger sample of the oldest-old in the NMES would be to integrate the sample designs for the NMES and the NHIS. The panel recognizes that the design and cost issues for such an approach are being carefully explored (National Center for Health Statistics, 1987a).

The panel design of the current National Medical Expenditure Survey will permit analysis of changes in utilization and expenditure patterns over the course of a year. However, to capture trends in utilization patterns in response to changes in delivery and payment systems over time, it will be necessary to repeat the survey every few years. Therefore, the panel reiterates its recommendation for a periodic national medical expenditure survey (Recommendation 8.3).

Relationship Between Health Status and Health Services Utilization

It is important to be able to relate the health and personal status characteristics of the elderly to their utilization of health services. Information on trends in the health status of the population could then be used to forecast changes in health services utilization patterns. The Medicare administrative records, or Medicare files, which contain utilization data on the elderly population age 65 and over who use the Medicare benefits to which they are entitled, are a useful source of data. Although there are an estimated 28 million Medicare beneficiaries in all (Young, 1985), only 75 percent of the elderly actually have Medicare claims on their behalf in any one year. The files are particularly useful in the area of hospitalization for acute episodes and other health services reimbursed by Medicare, but linkage to sources of information on total health services is needed.

The data files established to manage and monitor the Medicare program can be linked with records of the elderly in national surveys via items the two data bases have in common. Prominent among these surveys are the National Health Interview Survey, the planned National Medical Expenditure Survey, the National Nursing Home Survey (which includes a population component), and the Survey on Income and Program Participation. Performing such linkages would afford the opportunity to analyze health services utilization patterns of the elderly, derived from their Medicare files, in relation to their personal and health status characteristics, attitudes, and other pertinent socioeconomic and demographic information derived from interview surveys. Furthermore, such linked data sets would provide a rich source of longitudinal information on health services utilization by the elderly. This would make it possible to relate health status and other characteristics of the elderly to subsequent use of health services, and thereby to improve the capability of projecting future demands and costs for health services.

The type of linkage discussed is technically feasible and can be achieved without incurring the additional cost of collecting new data, although not without administrative costs. Although the Medicare files were established primarily to assist with administration and monitoring the Medicare program, the development of the Medicare Automated Data Retrieval System, as discussed in Chapter 8, will facilitate access to the Medicare files for research purposes (Lichenstein et al., no date). For a fuller discussion of the concept of data linkages and the methodology to achieve them, see Chapter 10; issues of confidentiality and access to records are also discussed in that chapter.

Recommendation 9.6: The panel recommends that (a) linkage with Medicare records be performed on a routine basis for persons age 65 and over who are respondents to population surveys that collect health data and (b) the Health Care Financing Administration and the National Center for Health Statistics explore linking the continuous National Health Interview Survey with the Medicare Automated Data Retrieval System, when the latter becomes operational.

Access to Care

In the two decades since the enactment of Medicare and Medicaid, impressive strides have been made in ensuring that more older Americans have access to the health care system. In addition, a backlog of long-neglected needs, especially among the elderly and the poor, was specifically addressed. For example, cataract operations that enable the elderly to improve their vision increased significantly following the introduction of Medicare. In 1982, the rate for this operation for both elderly men and women was three times that in 1965 (Rice, 1986).

Medicaid also has been successful in improving access to physician services for the population it covers—the poor and the "medically needy." Evidence suggests, however, that those near-poor not covered by Medicaid continue to lag well behind others in the use of services (Davis, 1985). Access to care still varies among subgroups of the population by income, race, and place of residence (President's Commission, 1983). Since the poor tend to be sicker than others, the higher medical care use rates among the poor do not necessarily indicate that they get more care given similar health status. An indicator of this is that poor persons of all ages, including the elderly, who report their health as fair or poor have significantly fewer physician visits than their counterparts in higher income groups (Kleinman et al., 1981). A major issue concerns the effect of changes in the deductible and coinsurance provisions of Medicare and in the eligibility and benefits under Medicaid on services utilized by the economically disadvantaged.

The growth of for-profit health care, the adoption of business-oriented approaches by health care providers, and the growth of competition in the medical care market may contribute to an unintended increase in the barriers to access to health care for our neediest citizens—many of whom are old. Changes in systems of care (HMOs, PPOs, etc.), increased emphasis on noninstitutional sources of care, and regulatory measures to contain costs (e.g., diagnosis-related groups for hospital reimbursement) are relevant for all segments of the aged and raise questions about many aspects of access, including what we mean by access and whether significant changes are occurring.

In a broad sense, access may be defined as the achievement of an appropriate match between need and utilization of services responsive to need. From this perspective, equity of access, then, may be said to exist "when services are distributed on the basis of need rather than as a result of structural or individual factors such as a family's income level, person's racial characteristics, or the distribution of physicians in an area" (Office of Technology Assessment, 1985a:96).

This leads to a close examination of factors that influence patterns of utilization of services among the elderly and changes that occur as a result of public and private initiatives in the health field. A useful framework for considering correlates of health care is to classify them as predisposing (e.g., social, demographic, psychological, and attitudinal characteristics of users and potential users of services), enabling (e.g., financial resources, availability of services, barriers to care), and need (objective or perceived need for care (see Andersen et al., 1983, for a brief review).

By now, these concepts are well established and a number of national population-based surveys have included items to measure access to care. Among these are the National Health Interview Survey (and its 1974 supplement on medical care availability and barriers to care), the Hispanic HANES (administered between 1982 and 1984), the Long-term Care Survey, the Longitudinal Study on Aging, the Survey of Income and Program Participation, and the National Medical Expenditure Survey and its predecessors. One national survey was designed explicitly for the purpose of measuring access to care among the general population—the National Survey of Access to Medical Care of the Center for Health Administration Studies of the University of Chicago, first conducted in 1970 and subsequently conducted in 1976 and in 1982 (see National Research Council, 1986 for a description).

The kinds of questions designed to measure access to care on the federal surveys include items concerning whether the respondent has a regular source of care and where he or she would go for care in case of need, the regularity or frequency of service utilization, the most recent visit or consultation with a health practitioner, queuing or waiting time to see health care providers, transportation time, and coverage or reimbursement for health care services. The Long-term Care Survey asks impaired elderly people directly about unmet needs for health care within the past month and why medical assistance has not been sought in the presence of unmet need. Perhaps the most comprehensive set of access questions to appear on a federal survey is found in the National Medical Expenditure Survey. This survey asks in detail about the usual source of care when ill, the use of a particular physician and dental office or clinic, the mode of transportation and length of time it takes to reach providers, waiting or queuing time to be seen, and insurance coverage and out-of-pocket costs for medical and health care.

Population-based surveys will continue to have a central role in identifying the impact of health care policies on access to services. This is particularly true for the continuous National Health Interview Survey, the periodic expenditure survey, the latest version of which is the National Medical Expenditure Survey, and the Longitudinal Study on Aging. Further, such population-based surveys can determine access problems of potentially vulnerable or high-risk segments of the population, such as the poor, the uninsured, specific racial and ethnic minorities, and the oldest-old. Surveys that include health status measures as well as access indicators make it possible to link adverse outcomes, such as the presence of health events that may reflect inadequate care or unmet need, with demographic and socioeconomic characteristics of individuals.

The National Health and Nutrition Examination Survey has the potential to be a particularly important vehicle for obtaining information on access to care in relation to health status. This is so because that survey, as its predecessors did, will collect objective indicators of health status derived from physical examinations and physiological and biochemical measurements along with information on health services received, which serve to determine unmet need whether it is recognized or unrecognized.

The elderly or segments of the elderly population may experience special or different problems or barriers in securing access to care than the remainder of the population. Not enough is currently known about the factors that affect utilization of health services by the elderly and about the access barriers experienced or perceived by older persons (Shapiro, 1986). Psychological factors or attitudes common among the present cohort of elderly, or particular subgroups of it, may play a role. The under-consumption of mental health services by the elderly relative to the prevalence of mental health problems among this population has been cited earlier in this chapter. In addition, demographic factors, educational level, and functional status, either mental or physical, may also affect the access characteristics of the elderly in special ways.

It is clear that while a great deal is known about access, there is need for a sharper focus on the status of access to care among different subgroups of the elderly and the effects on access of public policies in the health field.

Recommendation 9.7: The panel recommends that the National Center for Health Statistics, the National Center for Health Services Research and Health Care Technology, the National Institute on Aging, the National Institute of Mental Health, and other federal agencies that conduct or sponsor population-based surveys concerning the health of the elderly review the access-related items on existing and planned national surveys, whether privately or publicly sponsored, and work toward developing a standard set of access items that would be appropriate for use with elderly respondents in federally sponsored population surveys.

Population Subgroups

The Veteran Population The growing proportion of the elderly, particularly among men, who are veterans has been commented on extensively. The Veterans Administration is in a position to develop health-related information for the subgroup of veterans that utilize VA services. However, for a more complete understanding of patterns of care, health status, and access problems among veterans, it is necessary to turn to general population surveys.

The VA has conducted special surveys of veterans. Most of the surveys and data systems reviewed in this report identify whether or not the respondent or sampled person is a veteran, and these surveys have the advantage of providing trend data.

Recommendation 9.8: The panel recommends that the Veterans Administration take advantage of the information about veterans included in surveys and administrative records of other agencies to develop a data base for policy use.

The Poor and Near-poor Elderly The Medicaid program is the principal source of assistance to the poor and near-poor who seek health services and are not otherwise covered or eligible to receive such services. Although Medicaid is administered at the state level, national estimates of health services utilization by the Medicaid-eligible elderly who enroll in the program are available through the Medicaid Eligibility Quality Control system (MEQC). The purpose of the MEQC is to detect errors in eligibility determination and claims payments and misutilization by third-party payers. A sample of approximately 400,000 Medicaid enrollees in all states and territories (except Arizona, which did not participate in the Medicaid program at the time the sample was selected) is available for analysis of enrollee characteristics by service utilization characteristics. This data base shows promise of being developed into a useful data base of information on the poor and near-poor elderly (Adler, 1982).

The Medicaid Tape-to-Tape project, described in Chapter 8 also developed a data base, which, although limited to five states, provides utilization data on the poor, including the poor elderly who are enrolled in the Medicaid program in those states. For the panel's recommendation to the Health Care Financing Administration concerning elderly users of Medicaid services, see Recommendation 8.13 in Chapter 8.

The Rural Population A recent study of the National Research Council (1984) identified residents of rural areas as an underserved population and therefore likely to underutilize health care services relative to the utilization rates of other sectors of the population. The limited availability of health care providers, facilities, and services for health care in rural areas no doubt contributes to the underutilization of health care services by rural residents, including the rural elderly, according to that report. Information on the elderly's use of Medicare-covered services can be obtained from the Medicare Statistical System. Better data are needed, however, on comprehensive health services utilization and access to care on the part of the rural population generally and of the rural elderly in particular nationwide.

> **Recommendation 9.9:** The panel recommends that the National Center for Health Statistics and the National Center for Health Services Research and Health Care Technology take action to strengthen information regarding health services utilization and access to care among the rural population, by designing population-based surveys to include sufficiently large samples of the rural elderly population to provide suitably precise estimates for analytic evaluation of this population.

While the panel has concentrated on national data programs, it is important to recognize that two special studies, the Established Populations for Epidemiological Studies of the Elderly sponsored by the National Institute on Aging and the Epidemiologic Catchment Area, the research program conducted cooperatively by the National

Institute of Mental Health and academically based investigators, include panels of rural elderly people in selected states and localities (Iowa and North Carolina for the EPESE, and St. Louis, Missouri, and Durham, North Carolina, for the ECA). These two studies offer unique opportunities to document the health services utilization patterns of the rural elderly in these locations. The panel urges that these rural elderly panels be followed on a longitudinal basis.

10
Enhancing the Utility
of Statistical Systems

INTRODUCTION

The United States has a wide variety of data bases related to the health of the elderly—national data bases, state data bases, and some private data bases. The purpose of this chapter is to identify actions that can be taken to improve the utilization of existing data bases for policy analysis for the elderly. It addresses the third charge to the panel "to determine whether changes or refinements are needed in the statistical methodology used in health policy analysis or in the planning and administration of programs for the elderly and to recommend actions or further research." The recommendations in this chapter are much broader than those in earlier chapters because they generally concern all aging-related data bases rather than addressing a specific data system, a characteristic of recommendations in the previous chapters. A few of the previous recommendations are special cases of the broader recommendations in this chapter. This small amount of duplication is intended to help individuals concerned with improving data resources for a specific policy area, e.g., long-term care, since it might not otherwise be clear that a general recommendation would be important and relevant to a specific policy area.

The first section discusses issues pertaining to national data. This country has a large decentralized data system, at least 19 different agencies have responsibility for production and distribution of statistics related to one or more aspects of aging (Wallman, 1985:6):

Department of Agriculture
  Economic Research Service
  Food and Nutrition Service
Department of Commerce
  Bureau of the Census
Department of Health and Human Services
  Administration on Aging
  Alcohol, Drug Abuse, and Mental Health Administration
  Centers for Disease Control
  Health Care Financing Administration
  National Center for Health Services Research
  National Center for Health Statistics
  National Institute on Aging
  Office of Human Development Services
Office of the Assistant Secretary for Planning and Evaluation
  Social Security Administration
Department of Housing and Urban Development
  Office of Planning, Development, and Research
Department of Labor
  Bureau of Labor Statistics
  Employment and Training Administration
  Office of Pension and Welfare Benefit Programs
Department of the Treasury
Statistics of Income Division, Internal Revenue Service
Veterans Administration

Coordination, planning, and priority setting for these multiple data sources are required to make possible the analysis of data from multiple sources—a capability frequently required by policy makers. Several issues of coordination and planning are addressed, including content, coverage, data detail, uniform definitions, periodicity of data collection, and accessibility of data. The role of administrative records in policy making and research is also considered, as is the importance of designing surveys and administrative record systems in a manner that permits linkage between data systems.

The second section recognizes the importance of states both as sources and users of federal statistics and identifies several actions that could increase the value of federal statistics for use by states. Private sources of health-related information are reviewed briefly, primarily for the convenience of the reader who may wish to use the data but also to round out the panel's coverage of available data to ensure that no recommendations are made that would lead to duplication.

NATIONAL DATA

The panel believes that the federal government should place a very high priority on greater coordination and more consistent data policies among programs that produce statistics related to the elderly population. Currently, public policy is being developed in a context of major changes that affect the demand for and delivery of health services, as well as major changes in many other facets of policy that affect the lives of the elderly. Changes are likely to continue in the foreseeable future as budget constraints interact with population shifts and varying public demands. Such an atmosphere emphasizes the essential need to have adequate information to evaluate the effects of policy changes; unless attention is paid to ensure that as changes occur information is available to evaluate them, public policy will be made in a vacuum.

The issues that face this panel, though focusing on the health of the elderly, by necessity are interdisciplinary in nature. Issues of health cannot be considered without an understanding also of social, demographic, and economic characteristics and dynamics. As a result, although one agency may assume primary responsibility in providing a data series, in most circumstances several agencies will have a vested interest in developing data systems, preparing them for public use, and conducting various analyses.

These facets of the need for information on the elderly require a high degree of interagency cooperation and planning. It is with these concerns in mind that the panel makes its recommendations.

Background on Federal Statistical Policy

The U.S. federal statistical system has developed as a decentralized system: each department and major agency has one or more components that produce data related to the mission of the department. Responsibilities for the collection, processing, analysis, and dissemination of statistics are shared among program and statistical agencies. In the Department of Health and Human Services, for example, the National Center for Health Statistics is a major federal statistical agency, but several program agencies such as the Social Security Administration and the Health Care Financing Administration have large statistical programs based on administrative records, and the National Center for Health Services Research and Health Care Technology Assessment and the National Institutes of Health collect extensive statistical data as part of their research activities.

More than 60 years ago, a report prepared for the Congress by the Bureau of Efficiency noted (cited in Wallman, 1985:1)

> Practically every bureau in Washington collects or disseminates statistics of one kind or another; and there is much confusion in the public mind concerning the work done by the various offices. The statistics collected by the Government relate to nearly every aspect of our economic and social life. Statistics of agriculture begin with the seed and follow through to the marketing of the ripened product. Statistics of manufacturers extend from the mining of crude ore to the production of the manufactured article; those of commerce, from the lighting of rivers and harbors to the consumption of imported commodities; and those of social relationships from a mere enumeration of population to elaborate data regarding the incidence of disease.

Decades later, in 1985, the Office of Management and Budget identified more than 70 agencies having outlays of $500,000 or more for statistical activities in any of fiscal years 1984 to 1986 (U.S. Office of Management and Budget, 1985).

Although there have been many debates over the relative merits of maintaining a decentralized system (in contrast to a centralized statistical system such as exists in Canada and a number of European nations), that aspect of the system has not been changed. There are costs resulting from this decentralized structure related to ensuring the development of a comprehensive, nonduplicative, accurate, efficient, and accessible body of statistical information for the analysis of social, economic, and environmental issues. Problems in the data system are particularly likely to arise either when agencies share substantive responsibilities or when no single agency can be clearly identified as the most logical one to assume a responsibility. "For example, difficulties in ensuring the availability of a comprehensive and consistent body of data to explore the condition and problems of particular populations may arise when no single agency has lead responsibility for meeting information needs related to that population group" (Wallman, 1985:2).

Increasingly, in public policy forums, issues cut across substantive areas. These interrelationships mean that quantitative measures in one area are likely to be of significant use in related areas; data bases need to be combined, and consideration of possible relationships needs to be built into the processes of creating, expanding, and adjusting any new information systems.

As the complexity of the society, the economy, and the environment increases, the demands for data to better understand rapid changes also increase. Statistical agencies require a long planning horizon in order to have the lead time needed to collect and process data relevant to current issues. In the current fiscal environment, federal agencies need to undertake a serious long-term planning process, coordinated with planning of other statistical agencies, to address those areas for which social and policy change can be anticipated and formulated and for which data needs can be identified.

Legislative Authority for Statistical Policy

Office of Management and Budget

Since 1981, the legislative authority for the coordination and oversight of federal statistical programs has stemmed from The Paperwork Reduction Act of 1980 (44 U.S.C. S.3501-3520, in particular S.3504 (d)). That act establishes in the Office of Management and Budget (OMB) the Office of Information and Regulatory Affairs (OIRA) and charges the administrator of OIRA with, among other duties, statistical policy and coordination functions. The specific duties detailed in S.3504(d) are as follows:

The statistical policy and coordination functions of the Director shall include:

(1) developing long range plans for the improved performance of Federal statistical activities and programs;

(2) coordinating, through the review of budget proposals and as otherwise provided in this section, the functions of the Federal Government with respect to gathering, interpreting, and disseminating statistics and statistical information;

(3) developing and implementing Government-wide policies, principles, standards, and guidelines concerning statistical collection procedures and methods, statistical data classifications, and statistical information presentation and dissemination; and

(4) evaluating statistical program performance and agency compliance with Government-wide policies, principles, standards, and guidelines.

The act also assigns to OMB the responsibility to review and approve information collection requests (such as statistical surveys or administrative record systems) proposed by agencies. OIRA reviews such requests to prevent excessive burden on respondents, to prevent duplication of information collections among and within agencies, and to ensure adequate coverage of important issues (Wallman, 1985).

OIRA currently is not pursuing the goals of this legislation as aggressively as members of the statistical community and of the office itself might like. To meet the statistical policy mandate of the law, a statistical policy office was established in OIRA headed by the chief statistician. OIRA's initial authorization under the Paperwork Reduction Act of 1980 expired in 1983, after which the office and its activities were funded on a year-to-year basis from OMB's general appropriations (Council of Professional Associations on Federal Statistics, 1986). Since 1983, however, that office has had a staff of only six professionals to carry out the required functions for all statistical programs of the government. (By contrast, in previous years, the size of the statistical policy staff in the Office of Management and Budget reached as high as 69 in 1947, when the statistical programs of the federal government were substantially smaller and less complicated.)

As a result of staffing and fiscal constraints, the statistical policy office has had to be selective in the specific projects and tasks that it has initiated. The office is not currently focusing attention on statistics on the elderly; "active efforts to coordinate or improve the scope and quality of information on the elderly population are not being undertaken by OMB's Office of Information and Regulatory Affairs" (Wallman, 1985:9).

Congress recently passed The Paperwork Reduction Reauthorization Act of 1986, providing funding for OIRA for fiscal years 1987-1989 and amending the original act to correct problems surfaced during oversight hearings conducted by the House Committee on Government Operations and the Senate Committee on Governmental Affairs. A new requirement of the 1986 act with respect to the statistical policy and coordination functions is that the director of OMB include in an annual report to Congress (Council of Professional Associations on Federal Statistics, 1986:2):

(A)   a description of the specific actions taken, or planned to be taken, to carry out each function;

(B)   a description of the status of each major statistical program, includ-
        ing information on —
        (1)   any improvements in each such program;
        (2)   any program which has been reduced or eliminated; and
        (3)   the budget for each such program for the previous fiscal year
                and the fiscal year in progress and the budget proposed for
                the next fiscal year; and
(C)   a description and summary of the long-range plans currently in effect
        for the major Federal statistical activities and programs.

Congress is expected to continue to focus on OMB's implementation of its authorities. Recently the House Committee on Science
and Technology requested that the General Accounting Office inves-
tigate whether the OMB is "improperly and unnecessarily limiting
executive branch agencies in collecting, analyzing, and disseminating
information" (COPAFS, 1986:3).

Administration on Aging

A more specific legislative mandate for coordinating federal statistical programs specifically on the elderly population is in the Older
Americans Act of 1965, as amended, which assigns to the Administration on Aging (AOA) the responsibility to "gather statistics in
the field of aging which other federal agencies are not collecting,
and take whatever action is necessary to achieve coordination of
activities carried out or assisted by all departments, agencies, and
instrumentalities of the Federal Government with respect to the collection, preparation, and dissemination of information relevant to
older individuals." The act further assigns to the commissioner of
AOA the responsibility to advise, consult, and cooperate with the
head of each federal agency or department proposing or administering programs or services substantially related to the purposes of the
act and requires that each federal agency consult and cooperate with
the commissioner (Wallman, 1985).

The AOA has similar constraints to those of OIRA in terms
of resources available for these functions (only one individual is assigned to work on statistical issues, but the area of responsibility is
more narrowly delimited). The agency reviews plans for statistical
programs and publications of those few agencies that request such
review, but does not actively attempt to coordinate related programs
and issues among agencies.

With respect to statistics on the aging population, the most
notable problem resulting both from the constraints on resources
available for statistical policy oversight and coordination and from

the manner in which those resources are allocated is the lack of attention to identifying unmet data needs and to ensuring that such needs are met through modification of existing data systems or creation of new ones.

Informal Coordination Activities

Although only the OMB and the AOA have legislative authority for coordinating federal statistics on aging, other agencies have initiated activities to improve interagency coordination. Recently some progress has been made. On May 2, 1986, the National Institute on Aging and the Bureau of the Census cosponsored a Summit on Aging-Related Statistics. The purpose of the summit was to determine how the federal statistical system can provide the data needed to answer policy questions for an aging society in a cost-efficient manner. Participating agency directors prepared statements of their views on the vital issues regarding the elderly and agreed to establish an Interagency Forum on Aging-Related Statistics to encourage cooperation among the federal agencies in developing data on the older population (see Chapter 1 for more discussion of the forum). The agencies were commended for this initiative at the June 3, 1986, Senate hearings on statistical policy for an aging population, held by the Subcommittee on Energy, Nuclear Proliferation, and Government Processes of the U.S. Senate Committee on Governmental Affairs and the Subcommittee on Aging of the Committee on Labor and Human Resources. Congress recently appropriated funds for NIA for a second year of forum activities. Most of the funds are used for contracts with the Census Bureau and the NCHS to provide for intra-agency coordination of forum activities in these two agencies and for an annual report on these activities. A small portion of the funds is retained by NIA to carry out its forum responsibilities. A predecessor to the Forum on Aging-Related Statistics, an informal interagency group with a similar name (Forum for Statistics on Aging), was initiated by the Bureau of the Census in 1985 to exchange information, to coordinate the collection and tabulation of data on the elderly, and to identify data needs related to the elderly (Wallman, 1985). The early forum (now The Exchange) was also concerned with policy needs for data on the elderly and programmatic uses to which the data are put, but members were technical, professional agency staff rather than policy level staff.

The National Institute on Aging has recently established the

Subcommittee on Data Sources within the Interagency Committee on Research on Aging. The subcommittee has slightly different goals from those of the Census forum; in addition to serving as a means of exchanging information, the subcommittee attempts to assess how such sources have been influenced as research priorities have changed, to review data needs from the 1990 Census, and to provide agencies with feedback on concerns and priorities. The subcommittee is more concerned with how data sources relate to research issues than with the broader policy applications of data (Wallman, 1985).

Numerous examples exist of coordination of statistical programs at the initiative of one or two involved agencies. Agencies that are planning or changing a data collection will frequently attempt to notify other agencies that are known to have an interest; comment and review are also sought. Such efforts, however, tend to be fragmented and undependable. They are undertaken on an ad hoc basis and do not tend to play a consistent role in identifying duplication, excess burden, or data gaps.

COORDINATING, PLANNING, AND SETTING PRIORITIES FOR STATISTICS ON THE ELDERLY

In the area of statistics on the elderly population, coordination, oversight, and long-term planning are particularly important. As the number and proportion of elderly in the population increase, the needs of the population, from both the government and the private sector, will also increase, and, possibly more importantly, will change. If properly managed, the federal statistical system can provide information required for the society to cope with these changes. The data needs of agencies differ radically, but coordination of statistical programs on aging should be feasible. The panel commends the initiative taken by the NIA and the Census Bureau that led to the establishment of the Forum on Aging-Related Statistics—it is an important first step to improving interagency coordination of statistical programs related to aging—an activity that should be institutionalized.

> **Recommendation 10.1:** The panel recommends that a mechanism be provided for discussion and coordination of data needs, standardized definitions and classifications, priority identification, and production of data relating to an aging society.

The Forum on Aging-Related Statistics was recently established to function in this role. The panel recognizes that no single congressional committee has oversight of the statistical system, but the House Select Committee on Aging and the Senate Subcommittee on Aging have demonstrated strong interest in statistics on the elderly and might assume the oversight function for the activities of the forum.

Because little coordination is currently being undertaken, it is not possible to identify the magnitude of the cost effects of its absence. However, it should be clear that there are several areas in which the absence of coordination has direct effects that increase the inefficiencies of statistical programs. Failures of coordination, planning, and setting priorities lead to duplication of efforts, lesser sharing of data bases that might otherwise be of interagency use, unmet data needs, and inappropriate design of data bases for a broad array of data users. These effects alone imply that there are fiscal results of the lack of oversight. In addition, there are potentially serious effects with fiscal ramifications on other program agencies because of the lack of appropriate data for their policy planning and analysis.

Resources

In testimony before the Joint Economic Committee, U.S. Congress, April 17, 1986, James T. Bonnen placed strong emphasis on the deleterious effects of resource constraints on federal statistics (U.S. Congress, Senate, 1986b:304):

> We have already mortgaged the future of our capability to support informed decision in federal policy and elsewhere. Real resource constraints have led to major reductions in research activities in many statistical agencies. Personnel ceilings plus budget constraints have led to a failure to hire and hold a new generation of statisticians. Due to assaults on "useless bureaucrats" and a generally demeaning attitude toward federal employees, low morale and loss of many of the best people to early retirement and the private sector have affected many statistical agencies just as they have the rest of government. The long run has consistently been sacrificed to the short run. Where statistical leadership will come from 10 years from now, I shudder to think about. Sacrificing everything to the short run has reduced our ability to deal with the obsolescence of concepts that comes with change in markets, economic and social structure, institutions and new technologies.

This panel places high priority at this time on the allocation of resources to reverse the trends of the past few years that have reduced the number of appropriately qualified professionals in existing statistical agencies.

Decentralized Responsibility for Statistics on Aging

Not only are substantively different data sources located in a large number of separate agencies, but the agencies have interrelated responsibilities. For example, health-related statistics are produced by at least 12 of these agencies. In this decentralized environment, there are at least six issues of coordination and planning related to statistical surveys and administrative data on the elderly population that need to be addressed in an interagency context and by parties with the ability to influence the outcome of contested deliberations. The discussion of these issues here is limited to their relationships to statistical surveys; a subsequent section of the chapter discusses issues pertaining to administrative records.

Content

User agencies and policy analysts may have need for particular sorts of information that are not available from existing data sources and are not being planned for future data collections. Because primary data users are frequently not in close proximity to data producers, these needs may go unaddressed in the absence of an agency or other party responsible for identifying unmet data needs and determining means to meet them. Specific data gaps have been discussed in earlier chapters: these include longitudinal data on utilization and financing of health care, out-of-pocket expenses for medical and other care, alternative housing facilities, family support systems, types of long-term care, functional abilities, and chronic disease.

Coverage

Many of the ongoing surveys conducted by the Bureau of the Census are household surveys and do not include in their sampling frames those who do not live in households; they thus exclude the institutionalized population, which constitutes an important segment of the elderly population. For example, the nursing home population, which increases as a proportion of the population with each older age group and among women, is not included in many ongoing surveys, nor is the population of veterans in federal hospitals. Although specialized surveys are sometimes conducted to reach these groups that are not otherwise covered, the richness of content of any single survey is of necessity reduced.

Data Detail

The issue of data detail is, in some cases, related to the coverage issue discussed above. This problem, however, is more broadly defined to include all publications and other forms of data dissemination that do not include adequate detail on special populations. As the elderly population increases in size and as a proportion of the total population, it becomes increasingly important to know more about specific groups within that population. For different purposes, additional detail may be needed on the oldest-old, five-year age groups among the elderly, women, minorities, those with health problems, the poor elderly, or other specialized populations. Sometimes surveys do not include enough cases of particular subpopulations in their sample, and the issue is one of coverage. Larger overall samples or specialized oversampling may be required. In other cases, information that is issued in aggregate form may simply not include enough detail in the aggregated groups to identify those subpopulations; the problem in this circumstance is one of data presentation for the needs of data analysts.

The rapidly changing distribution of the aged population requires a reexamination of the sampling frames for studies collecting data on which future plans for people of age 65 and over depend. Table 10.1 shows the projected sharp increase in the total elderly population and the substantial increases among the very old over the period 1980 to 2010.

Surveys designed in the 1980s for a sample of the entire population may include too small a number of the age group 65 and over to answer many questions for detailed age subgroups of this population. Numbers in the age group 85 and over may be especially deficient for the description of the characteristics of the oldest-old.

The panel urges that the sample design for population surveys be matched to the major policy questions to be addressed. Sample sizes should be large enough to permit accurate estimation for persons in age-specific subgroups of the older population through further disaggregation of data. Subgroups of interest include those near the

TABLE 10.1 Size of the Older Population 1980-2010 (in thousands)

Age	1980	1990[a]	2000[a]	2010[a]
Total	25,549	31,697	34,921	39,195
65-69	8,782	9,996	9,096	11,703
70-74	6,798	8,039	8,581	8,615
75-79	4,794	6,260	7,295	6,782
80-84	2,935	4,089	5,023	5,544
85-89	1,520	2,157	3,025	3,756
90+	720	1,156	1,901	2,795

[a]Bureau of the Census Middle Level Projections.

Source: Serow and Sly (1985: Tables 1 and 22).

age of eligibility for Medicare and Social Security (both pre- and postretirement groups), and the oldest-old.

The panel recognizes that it may be costly to screen extra cases to identify members of the age group 65 and over and that there are costs attached to increased sample sizes. Nonetheless, we urge that consideration be given to this issue at the survey design stage. The panel is not advancing a specific sample size for the population age 65 and over, but we urge that agencies planning surveys reexamine the question of adequacy of the sample for analysis purposes. We recognize that the adequacy of the sample depends on the nature of the analytic methods being considered.

Uniform Definitions, Concepts, and Classifications

Surveys (and administrative record systems) that collect related information do not always do so using the same definitions and concepts, even though doing so would increase the usefulness of each of the information sources involved. The importance of standard definitions was illustrated in the chapter on long-term care.

In the data collection stage, categories used are not always the same; as a result information from different surveys may not be comparable. In later stages of data processing, differences in classifications may further reduce comparability. Uniformity is required for purpose of compatibility and could, with proper foresight and interest in the planning stages, be achieved.

The single most useful standard that agencies could adopt is to provide information for standard age categories in publications and public use files. In addition, the panel urges that agencies include the date of birth in public use files whenever possible. This is particularly important for the elderly, since they frequently report age incorrectly.

Recommendation 10.2: The panel recommends that agencies that collect and disseminate data on the total population or administrative data by age: (1) use 5-year age groups for the publication of data up to age 90 and larger intervals thereafter, except when limited by privacy or confidentiality regulations and (2) provide data on geographic areas, income, and other economic characteristics in the greatest level of detail consistent with the protection of confidentiality.

Issues of confidentiality and privacy are frequently invoked as the rationale for limiting the levels of geographic detail or the detailed breakdowns provided on specific data items. Confidentiality restrictions in these cases can severely limit the utility of the data. It is clear that confidentiality must be respected to safeguard the integrity of the statistical system and to honor commitments to respondents. It is equally clear that confidentiality should not be used as an excuse for withholding disaggregated data.

Periodicity

The frequency with which surveys are conducted, or periodicity, as well as the scheduling of the data collections is a matter that clearly affects the timeliness of the data and the comparability among data sources. Although a data-producing agency may allocate limited resources by reducing the periodicity of a survey, this may have severe consequences for policy analysts. A recent example of this was the National Nursing Home Survey, which had originally been planned to be conducted every three years; eight years lapsed between the last two such surveys. Little was known in the intervening period about changes in this rapidly increasing subpopulation that consumes an increasing proportion of total medical expenditures—a time period during which the major health issue confronting Congress was control of medical expenditures. Moreover, when surveys are conducted less frequently than annually, it is sometimes of concern whether the timing of the data collection itself is synchronized with other surveys or record systems since policy analysts may need data from multiple sources for the same time period.

> **Recommendation 10.3:**   The panel recommends that greater emphasis be placed on establishing and maintaining the periodicity of population surveys. The periodicity should be established with due consideration of seasonality, secular trends, the frequency of changes in policy, the importance of the issues addressed in public policy, and the timing of related data collections.

Data Access

Although data producers in the federal government have placed greater attention in recent years on producing public use tapes and providing greater access to data, more attention still needs to be paid to this area. Without timely access to data, researchers gain little from the fact that a data base has been collected and processed. The systematic development of a plan to ensure public access to published reports and to microdata files is a necessary part of the development of any data program. The data collection agencies frequently have insufficient research staff to fully utilize data bases, and priority should be placed on providing outside researchers with access.

When there are issues of confidentiality of data, such as may arise with the development of linked data bases, public access is a more complicated problem. Even so, there are precedents for providing access in innovative ways, such as enabling outside researchers to conduct research within the agency that has produced the files.

The Office of Management and Budget on December 12, 1985, issued Circular No. A-130, Management of Federal Information Resources. The purpose of this circular is to establish policy for the management of all federal information resources, providing procedural and analytic guidelines for policy implementation. With respect to data access, the first policy the circular establishes is that agencies shall "create or collect only that information necessary for the proper performance of agency functions and that has practical utility, and *only after planning for its processing, transmission, dissemination, use, storage, and disposition.*" This circular was issued by the Office of Information and Regulatory Affairs and establishes the interest and authority of that office to review and monitor the dissemination of data.

The circular indicates that agencies' primary interest is not necessarily in disseminating information products and services, but rather that they must attend to the legal requirements to do so, to the relationship between issuing products and services and the agencies' missions, and to public need for the products. In addition, agencies have an obligation to make data available to those who have a reasonable ability to acquire the information, in a manner cost-effective for the government, and, whenever possible, to recover the costs of dissemination.

Data access has, in general, been a weak point in the development of federal data bases on health and health policy. This area must be improved if researchers are to be able to conduct studies in a timely manner. The panel recognizes that the new OMB circular addresses many of these issues, but it also recognizes that the manner in which the circular is implemented remains to be determined. We believe that agencies must adequately plan for public access to their data bases and that a high priority must be placed on timely and complete access. Not only should access be provided to files created for the purpose of providing statistical information, but it should also be improved for statistical files created from administrative record systems.

> **Recommendation 10.4:** The panel recommends that the plans of a federal agency for the creation or continuation of a data system should include a plan for issuance of publications and public use tapes following its creation or updating. The plan should include explicit procedures for disseminating the data and should provide for widespread access and timely, thorough, and accurate data dissemination.

In addition to the timely dissemination of public use tapes, provision should be made for archiving such data bases to maximize their utilization by nongovernmental researchers and analysts.

> **Recommendation 10.5:** The panel recommends the continued support and development of (a) aging-related archives of research data, such as the National Archive of Computerized Data on Aging at the University of Michigan and (b) provision of technical support for users.

Confidentiality

"The essence of statistical confidentiality . . . is that statistics released by the collecting agency or researcher cannot be related to data provided by or about an identifiable respondent. This principle is considered to be a cornerstone of statistical policy" (President's Reorganization Project for the Federal Statistical System, 1981:200).

High-quality data can be obtained only when the confidentiality of the respondent can be convincingly guaranteed by the data collection and processing agencies. In the past, the statistical policy office of OMB has had a long history of placing a high priority on ensuring that statistical data are kept confidential. Some data series are kept confidential until scheduled release times. More relevant for the considerations of this panel, however, is the strict maintenance of confidentiality of microdata records. The Bureau of the Census and the National Center for Health Statistics are the only statistical agencies that now have a statutory basis to ensure the confidentiality of their records. Although other agencies, such as the Bureau of Labor Statistics, have no statutory basis to guarantee the confidentiality of their data collections, they do so on their own, and because of their effectiveness in honoring that guarantee they have obtained a high level of voluntary reporting.

Another important consideration for the maintenance of the confidentiality of records, however, arises from the need for data sharing among statistical and administrative agencies. Data sharing can reduce respondent burden, duplication, and the fiscal budgets of statistical agencies. The types of data sharing for which this is the case include, for example, sharing of sampling frames for specialized subpopulations and sharing of statistical or administrative data bases for statistical or exact matching. Although the context of such sharing should always be to produce statistical, aggregate information from combined data bases, when more than one agency is involved, even if both are statistical agencies, problems may arise in the sharing of records. If one agency has an umbrella legislative guarantee of confidentiality and another has no such guarantee, the first is likely to be reluctant to share its data. Agencies without such legislative authority that have nevertheless guaranteed their respondents confidentiality may also be reluctant to share data, even for statistical purposes.

Efforts to establish a broad cover of confidentiality guarantees for the entire federal statistical system have in the past been met with some skepticism. Many believe that the right of individuals to privacy, to provide what information they wish with full knowledge about how that information will be used, should be paramount in consideration of these issues. The issue is not only that individuals have been promised confidentiality in the statistical sense for the information they provide, but also that they have provided informed consent when they have provided that information. Opponents have expressed concern that widespread data sharing could lead to the creation of large-scale data banks that would contain substantial amounts of information about different facets of individuals' lives or the characteristics of businesses, even though respondents would never have provided all that information to one government agency. Concern for the potential abuse of such a system has weighed more heavily in the minds of some than the conveniences of being able to reduce respondent burden and budgets.

Administrative Records

There are two major sources for developing information on the elderly—surveys of individuals that have the capacity for including characteristics on a personal basis such as health status or demographic characteristics and administrative records that have information relative to an individual's participation in a government program in conjunction with certain characteristics of the individual. Surveys are based on well defined sampling frames and are generalizable to well-defined population groups, whereas administrative records provide information only for individuals using a service or selected into a program. Administrative records are not a substitute for surveys but a complementary source for some types of statistics on certain subgroups of the population.

Administrative records are typically produced by agencies with direct programmatic responsibilities as a by-product of their administrative or regulatory procedures, sometimes for program analysis, but more frequently for monitoring individual cases within specific programs. As a result, the data in these records tend to be limited to data required for administration of the program. Additional socioeconomic and demographic background information so frequently essential for analysis is typically lacking.

The use of administrative records for statistical purposes has increased substantially over the past decade. Administrative records serve as an attractive source of data for some purposes. Often they are the only available source of specific information needed for policy analysis. In addition, they can frequently provide data for small geographic areas or small subpopulations, while minimizing respondent burden and data collection costs. Problems arise in using such records because they frequently cover only limited populations or limited substantive detail, access is inhibited by law or administrative procedure, data quality is not always consistent (e.g., financial data may be accurate while health records are incomplete or unreliable), and records may not be kept for the same units that are needed for statistical analysis.

In some cases, however, administrative records may be a superior source of information to respondent-provided information. When data are available on records, they may be more accurate if they are associated with the actual operation of the administrative program for which the records are being kept. In such cases the use of records is desirable, even when linkages must be made to other data sources to complete data sets for statistical analysis.

There are costs and operational problems associated with making administrative records suitable for statistical purposes or with linking them with other statistical data bases to obtain more complete information on the units of analysis. However, such costs and the work required to process the records for statistical use may be much less than that associated with new data collections to obtain the same information.

Active statistical policy coordination and oversight is needed to enhance the use of administrative records for statistical purposes. Data policies can facilitate the innovative production of data, ensure confidentiality of information on both administrative and statistical record systems, encourage the greater use of administrative records, ensure maximum data quality, ensure that resources are made available for upgrading the quality and content of record systems, and stimulate interagency deliberations as needed.

The panel recognizes that there are many problems inherent in increasing the use of administrative records, but we believe that these problems can be addressed and, in many cases, overcome. In cases of statistical uses of administrative records, particular care must be taken to safeguard traditional assurances of confidentiality of statistical data. The statistical agencies, to secure their own data collections, must take special care in how they handle these records and how they share data with program agencies.

Recommendation 10.6:   The panel recommends that greater use be made of administrative records as a source of statistical information on the elderly. To facilitate this goal, special attention should be paid to designing data tapes, including public use tapes, from administrative record systems to make them more useful and accessible to policy analysts and researchers to the extent feasible within confidentiality constraints.

Data Linkages

Related to, but separable from, the issues of administrative records are issues of linkages between data sets. Such linkages can be accomplished either through matches of records on the same individuals from different data bases, known as exact matches, or through matches of records on different individuals who are identified as identical or similar in important respects, known as statistical matches. Statistical matching should be used as a last resort, and then used with great caution. Both types of matches serve to provide a broader set of data on individual cases by merging two or more data sets that supply different sets of characteristics. There are specialized problems associated with each type of linkage. In addition to the technical problems, however, there are also broad problems of statistical policy associated with the linking of records from different agencies and of administrative and survey records.

The power of linked records lies in the ability to expand available information at the microdata level without undertaking new data collections. The process draws on the strengths of administrative records when they are turned to as a source of possibly more accurate data than could be obtained in an interview setting. Linkage of administrative data with survey data can also enrich the administrative data system.

The increased use of data linkages can be enhanced by more active coordination among agencies that need such data as well as among those that have the data bases to be matched. The function of coordination and oversight in this case is very similar to the role discussed above for the use of administrative records. It revolves around ensuring confidentiality and quality, identifying appropriate content areas, assisting in interagency deliberations, and reducing respondent burden and fiscal costs.

Recommendation 10.7: The panel recommends greater use of data base linkages as a source of statistical information on the elderly. Unless there are confidentiality limitations, barriers to linking data systems should be removed. Resources should be made available to increase the flexibility of these systems.

Enhancement of National Surveys

This report includes a number of recommendations to enhance surveys that are relevant to all agencies that collect data about the elderly. In addition, a large number of recommendations have been made to augment specific health surveys. Many surveys other than health surveys are related to the health of the elderly, such as the Retirement History Survey, the American Housing Survey, and the Survey of Income and Program Participation. We have singled out the last survey for discussion since it has the potential for providing longitudinal data on the health of the elderly and for relating health to income.

Survey of Income and Program Participation

The Survey of Income and Program Participation, first administered in October 1983, is a nationally representative household survey that provides detailed longitudinal information on income, living arrangements, disability, assets and liabilities, government transfer program eligibility and participation, pension coverage, taxes, and many other characteristics of individuals. Each February a new panel of about 15,000 households enters the survey. Members of each panel are interviewed every 4 months over a period of 32 months; the longitudinal design of the survey, which provides 8 interviews for each household, allows for the study of changes in characteristics. In addition to the core of labor force and income questions, fixed topical modules are administered periodically during the survey. SIPP can be especially useful in analyses relating economic status to health questions.

In the first interview of the 1984 SIPP, there were over 11,000 sample cases of people age 55 and over; their distribution by age group is shown in Table 10.2.

The sample is too small for statistically reliable analyses by age groups beyond age 75 and over. It would be desirable to augment the SIPP sample of the population over age 65 periodically, e.g., every five years. It would not be necessary to oversample the population age 65 and over in all panels. Oversampling could be facilitated by using Social Security or Medicare records to identify additional persons age 75 and older.

TABLE 10.2 First Interview of the 1984 Survey of Income and Program Participation (unweighted counts)

Age	Total
55-64	5,116
65-74	3,880
75-84	1,856
85+	446

Recommendation 10.8: The panel recommends that the Survey of Income and Program Participation sample be augmented at the beginning of each five-year interval to provide suitably precise estimates of characteristics for groups ages 75-84 and 85 and over.

One of the topical modules used in SIPP is on health and disability. This module includes extensive questions on health status, need for help in activities of daily living, person providing assistance, type of disability and disability-caused limitations on kind and amount of work. Other modules cover topics such as education and work history, pension plan coverage, retirement plans and expectations, marital history, fertility history, taxes, asset holdings, and employee benefits (the last module has little relevance for the elderly). The utility of the data collected in SIPP might be increased by targeting specific modules to appropriate subgroups of the population. It would be possible to obtain longitudinal data on health and disability of the elderly by administering the health and disability module a second time to those over age 65 instead of the employee benefits module. This substitution would require somewhat more complex procedures for interviewers, but it should be feasible.

Recommendation 10.9: The panel recommends that, in administering the Survey of Income and Program Participation, the Bureau of the Census replace the topical module on employee benefits with the health and disability module for one wave for those of age 65 and over so the latter module is used twice, ideally at a two-year interval.

The Bureau is exploring the possibility of matching administrative records from the Social Security Administration with the SIPP records to provide additional information on the elderly. Records being considered for matching include summary earnings records, benefit records, and Medicare records.

FEDERAL-STATE DATA ISSUES

Background

Since the beginning of American federalism both the development and the administration of social policy has depended on the joint efforts of the federal and state governments. Paralleling the cooperative federal nature of policy implementation itself, the collection and preparation of the data necessary to monitor and evaluate social policies and programs also depend on a variety of federal-state cooperative activities.

The states, as well as the several agencies of the federal government, are both producers and consumers of data. While states may be the greatest consumers of their own, largely administrative, data, the importance of the crossover linkages between federal and state agencies cannot be overemphasized. That is especially true of the area of national vital statistics, in which the states are the key suppliers of what become national data files.

Simultaneously, the bloc grant context of New Federalism has placed significantly increased importance upon a variety of state-government-directed intrastate resource allocation, planning, and monitoring activities. That is, the implementation of federal (as well as state) programs is increasingly undertaken through the allocation of resources by state governments to targeted populations identified through county and other substate units.

For example, through the Older Americans Act, state governments receive federal funds in support of a broad range of nutrition and social services. Federal law requires that the state governments allocate these funds through an intrastate funding formula to planning and service areas across the state in such a way that funds are targeted to those elderly in "greatest economic or social need." Since these planning and service areas are *aggregations of counties*, age-specific county-level population data required for assessing need are a crucial element of this planning and resource allocation process.

Consequently, the federal supply of national population statistics, disaggregated to county and other substate levels, represents an increasingly important—and irreplaceable—source of data. It is against this backdrop of the necessary cooperative relationship between federal and state data sources and data needs that the panel directs attention to the following six issues.

Vital Statistics and Data on Mortality

Vital statistics representing data on births, deaths, marriages, divorces, and other demographic indicators, constitute a critical national resource, yet represent primarily a data collection activity on the part of state governments. As part of the Vital Statistics Cooperative Program, states collect their vital statistics data and subsequently make them part of the national data system through contracts with the National Center on Health Statistics. Under this program, the NCHS, in conjunction with appropriate state agencies, develops definitions and standards for state data collection and also provides technical assistance to the state agencies.

Of special interest to an aging society is detailed information concerning the distribution of causes of death. While "old age" may have been an acceptable designation of the cause of death in an earlier era, both the technical capacity and the greater need for more detailed mortality statistics suggests the importance of more focused analysis of death certificates and the reporting of mortality statistics. The analysis of mortality within an aging population represents, among other factors, an important dimension of the epidemiology of the health of that population. A recent NCHS study, for example, reported that nearly 75 percent of the death certificates studied had more than one condition listed and 15 percent had more than four conditions listed (National Center for Health Statistics, 1984a). Up to 20 conditions reported on the death certificate are coded. With greater detail in the reporting and enumeration of deaths, it will be possible to better identify patterns of morbidity and mortality by region, state, and substate areas, as well as by age, sex, and race. The identification of such patterns are important for both scientific analyses, and policy and program decisions.

The NCHS has released tapes of multiple causes of death for the years 1968-1983 to encourage their use by analysts and researchers. The Multiple Causes of Death Data Files are good sources of data for research purposes, but they are used by only a few researchers.

Recommendation 10.10: The panel commends the National Center for Health Statistics for developing the Multiple Causes of Death Data Files and for preparing public use tapes of those files. The panel recommends that the Center develop an outreach program to promote their use.

The death certificate contains an item on whether an autopsy was performed, but because of the legal requirements for prompt filing of death certificates, autopsy information even for the small percentage (13 percent) of the deaths autopsied is not always used in the preparation of the cause of death statement. The panel urges that NCHS and state vital statistics offices cooperate in efforts to improve the quality and completeness of the medical certification through better training of physicians, and through query programs, with emphasis on augmenting the certification by appending autopsy information when available.

Disability Statistics

While most older persons live in their own homes and are not constrained in most of their daily activities by disability, knowledge of the distribution of disability of an aging population is especially important. A broad range of both state and federal health and social service programs is dependent on knowledge of such disability statistics for the allocation of resources and the monitoring of the programs. While the 1980 census included a disability item, it was notably limited for use with respect to the older population because its context was that of employment-connected disability. A number of federal agency surveys include specific measures of health and disability, yet most such surveys provide only national estimates or state estimates without statistical detail at the substate level. By contrast, health policy planning and scientific analyses undertaken for an aging society require detailed age and age-sex distributions of disability.

Since a variety of health and social service programs respond to the varying needs of different disabilities, neither age data per se nor data on institutionalization are an acceptable substitute for precise disability data per se. Furthermore, as noted previously, given that state agencies have increased programs that provide social services to the elderly and disabled, state and substate disability data are increasingly important tools for planning, evaluation, and analysis.

The panel recognizes that in the continuing planning for the 1990 census, the director of the Bureau of the Census is giving emphasis to the development and testing of items that will provide detailed measures of functional disability sensitive to the needs of an aging population.

> **Recommendation 10.11:** The panel recommends that age-sensitive disability items be included in the 1990 census and that estimates for states and major civil subdivisions, by age, be tabulated and published.

Age Detail

The traditional social definition of "old" as age 65—tied to the long-standing age of full benefits eligibility under Social Security—appears to influence the reporting of many state and federal age distributions. Both demographically and in terms of policy, it is evident that the population is aging, that there are increasing numbers of persons living to older ages, and consequently there is a fundamental need to change the norms of statistical data reporting for a broad range of variables and indicators. And as noted, state planning requires increasingly sophisticated age data, including more detailed description of the population over age 65. It is imperative that the major statistical agencies of the federal government, not just the specialized age-related or health-related agencies, routinely report detailed age data beyond age 65, so that the requisite planning and analytic data sets will then become more broadly available. For purposes such as assessing the potential impact of changes in the age for eligibility for Medicare or Social Security, distributions by single year of age are needed.

> **Recommendation 10.12:** The panel recommends that in publishing decennial census data for geographic subareas of the country, the Bureau of the Census provide age, age-sex, and age-sex-race distributions beyond age 65. Whenever feasible, distributions by single year of age should be made available. At a minimum, such age detail should be made available at the county level by 5-year age intervals through age 85. Furthermore, within the normal constraints of the protection of individual privacy, the Bureau of the Census should make a broad range of population data available with age detail beyond age 65 for states, counties, and other sub-state areas.

Dissemination of Age-detailed Substate Data

Throughout this discussion two themes have been emphasized: the need for data to be made available at the substate level and the need for greater age detail in population and vital statistics data. One valuable source of such data is the State Data Center in each state, whose responsibility is to process census data tapes for a variety of data users. (Parallel organizations, such as the Association of State and Territorial Health Officers, also serve as information sources in this regard.)

State Data Centers exhibit substantial variation in the kinds of data and data services they supply, some having developed into national wholesalers of census and market research data, while others having defined a fairly narrow set of technical services. A further limitation of State Data Centers can be seen from the perspective of the health and social policy analyst who requires detailed age data from across the country. As one might expect, for example, even when the State Data Centers do prepare intercensal substate estimates of the size and status of the older population—and not all states do—they use a variety of different methodologies in the computation of those estimates.

A complementary source of age-detailed substate data is reflected in another existing data dissemination model: the *County and City Data Book* represents an especially rich collection of substate data that has been produced in printed form by the Census Bureau for many years. Its value is enhanced by the fact that it includes, in addition to population census data: a selection of vital statistics; housing data; education and crime statistics; data on poverty, employment, and unemployment; statistics on doctors, nurses, dentists, hospitals, and nursing homes; and substate information on Social Security and Medicare, including dollars distributed and persons involved. The sheer variety of the variables included provides both state and local officials as well as researchers with a unique capacity to understand and explore the population and environment of the American people at the local level, where an increasing amount of planning and service delivery are taking place.

The value of the *County and City Data Book* as a state and substate planning and analytic tool was enhanced when the Census Bureau made the collection available in computer-readable formats. In the context of the microcomputer revolution of the past decade, it is especially noteworthy that in 1984 the Census Bureau began distributing this data base on microcomputer diskette, thereby making it more accessible to a much broader array of state planning agencies.

Given the general value of the collection of data in the *County and City Data Book*, its utility for an aging population is unfortunately limited. The old age variable itself is limited to "percent 65+," and none of the other important indicators of the health and wealth of the population is presented for different age categories. Given the availability of such age detail throughout the other parts of the census data system, in addition to the widespread utility of the city-county data base and the demonstrated ease of access to it via its recent diskette dissemination format, this data base should be further developed for use in the context of an aging population.

> **Recommendation 10.13:** The panel recommends that the director of the Census Bureau develop plans to produce an enhanced, age-detailed *County and City Data Book* data set. Consistent with standards for protecting the privacy of individuals in small statistical areas, county and city data representing age detail, by five-year age categories through age 85 whenever possible, should be assembled for the range of population, health, poverty, employment, race and ethnicity, and other variables currently included in the *County and City Data Book*. It is recommended that such a data set be assembled and made available using the 1990 census and related data collections and distributed in both printed and machine-readable formats (computer tape and microcomputer diskette formats) on a timely basis.

Timely Substate Data

Health planners in state, county, and local areas require information on the size and distribution of the elderly population in order to budget for community health services, hospital beds, nursing homes, and other related services. Decennial figures from the Census of Population and Housing are soon outdated. The sample sizes of the Current Population Survey or the Survey of Income and Program Participation are too small to provide small-area estimates of characteristics of the elderly population.

In 1976, Congress authorized a mid-decade census in the year 1985 and every 10 years thereafter by amending Title 13 of the United States Code-Census (U.S. Congress, Senate, 1976). No census was taken in 1985; the earliest possible date for a quinquennial census is now 1995. With the rapid growth and internal migration of the population, health planners need reliable and timely estimates of the population by age, race, sex, and income level and in geographic detail to the minor division level. The mid-decade census would fill this need for all jurisdictions. The panel recognizes that the cost of the mid-decade census requires justification far beyond that which can be supplied by health planners but views this as an important need that should be taken into consideration.

Social Service Statistics

Since 1965 the federal and state governments have supported an array of social services, including nutrition programs, for the elderly through the Older Americans Act. From the beginning, but especially since 1973, these programs have reflected the principles of federalism, in that national funding, guidelines, and priorities have been implemented by State Units on Aging and a within-state network of Area Agencies on Aging. Data collections that represent services provided, clients served, and dollars allocated and spent therefore reflect both the national guidelines and priorities and the state and local implementation of these national mandates.

Despite the fact that these nutrition and social service programs reflect their state and local implementations, the statistical data that describe the programs represent important national data, since nutrition and social programs are significant factors in maintaining the health and independence of the older population. Since 1978 the National Association of State Units on Aging (NASUA) and the National Association of Area Agencies on Aging (N4A), professional associations representing the administrators of the state and area agencies, have been supported by the Administration on Aging to collect budgetary, client, and service delivery data reflecting the several programs of the Older Americans Act. These data are collected on a continuing basis; periodic and annual updates are crucial given the changing nature of both the older population and the service programs that serve them.

In many cases the program data can be matched with demographic and other national data, since the planning areas served by the Area Agencies on Aging are aggregations of counties. This merging of program and demographic data sets offers a valuable opportunity to monitor and assess changes in the aging population and the effectiveness of social programs in helping to maintain the health of the aging population.

While the panel does not make a specific recommendation in this regard, the importance of maintaining this unique data collection is acknowledged.

Private Data Bases

Very few private data bases in the health area are publicly available, and there is no central repository enumerating all private data bases. Data bases are therefore examined for the industries considered most pertinent to health policy for an aging population, namely hospitals, nursing homes, HMOs, hospices, private insurance companies, and professional associations.

Hospital Data

Within the hospital industry, their trade association, the American Hospital Association (AHA) collects data on a regular basis. Four primary instruments are utilized at various intervals: the Annual Survey of Hospitals, the National Hospital Panel Survey, the Survey of Medical Rehabilitation Hospitals and Units, and the Survey of Medical Staff Organization. The data collected by these surveys focus primarily on facility characteristics (numbers of beds, medical staff organization, character of overall facilities), health resources (types of services within facility, types of resources connected to facility, quality and training of medical/health staff), financial data, and services utilization.

No new surveys are being planned, but as the industry and relevant technology evolve, the surveys are modified to meet data needs. The AHA makes all of its data bases publicly available in either tape or hard copy, at a charge and within the limits of confidentiality.

Nursing Home Data

Data collection for the nursing home industry is less well organized. One of the primary obstacles to comprehensive data collection within this sector is the lack of standardized definitions for what actually constitutes a nursing home and what actual services fall within a particular colloquial definition. Given the broad facility licensure authority within each state, it is not feasible to collect comparable data across the industry.

Currently, at least one trade association, the American Health Care Association (AHCA) is collecting data from its membership. The data are limited to numbers of facilities within a region, occupancy rate, ongoing growth of industry, and financial expenditure/reimbursement information. Currently, these data are available only to association members and have been used to support articles in trade publications and lobbying efforts. The AHCA plans to expand its data collection efforts to include services utilization and opinions on current issues and has indicated that the data could be made available within the applicable strictures of confidentiality.

Health Maintenance Organization Data

A different arena, one that has undergone substantial growth and change, is the health maintenance organization industry. Particularly because of the uneven growth in enrollment, services, and utilization trends, this industry also lacks a set of standardized definitions with which to conform any potential data base. Because of the unique reimbursement system between HCFA and HMOs, it has become nearly impossible to elicit cooperation from HMOs vis-a-vis services rendered. This is due partly to the unique record-keeping systems in HMOs, and in part to the proprietary nature of the information.

Notwithstanding these obstacles, the Group Health Association of America (GHAA), a trade association for HMOs, has undertaken a major project to develop and implement a uniform data collection system for HMOs. To date, modules of tables based on items with standard definitions have been developed and are being pretested for statistics on enrollment and marketing, health services delivery, finances, and health care purchases. Completion and implementation of this project could take several years. Given that GHAA's membership organizations represent a large majority of all HMO enrollment, that the system design group is composed of a broad spectrum of HMOs nationwide, and that GHAA plans to make the data base available to the public within strict confidentiality guidelines, the project has the potential of generating a useful data base.

Hospice Data

An industry that deals with the aging population as a part of its clientele is hospice. Because of its relative youth as an industry, very little has been done to develop a publicly available private data base.

The National Hospice Organization publishes an annual membership directory and the Hospice Association of America is developing a membership survey to ascertain information from providers, including field of service, types of personnel, type of facility, and whether associated with another health care unit, numbers of patients served, and financing/reimbursement data. The data base from this survey is still being developed; data will not be available before summer 1988.

Commercial Health Insurance Data

The Health Insurance Association of America, whose membership represents 95 percent of the commercial health insurance business, currently is involved in three major data collection efforts. The Survey of Hospital Semi-Private Room Charges is currently available to the public at reproduction cost. It contains average room cost for responding hospitals by zip code. The Prevailing Health Care Charges System is available to members and certain research associations only. The data are tabulated by zip code and are available at reproduction cost. The *Source Book of Health Insurance Data* (a compilation of Health Insurance Association of America data and data collected by government and other organizations) is an annual publication available to the public without charge.

It seems reasonable to ask why there are no statistical data produced as by-products from the large number of health insurance providers, HMOs, etc., just as there are from Medicare and the Social Security system.

Two elements that are fundamental elements of a statistical system to assess utilization of medical care are lacking in the data collected by insurance companies: (1) a population base, in which every insured individual is separately identified—the population data provide the denominator for a ratio and (2) an individual record of use of service and its nature and costs or charges or both, which can be used individually or combined for subgroups of the population (e.g., age groups or race-ethnic groups) as the numerator of the ratio.

The rate structure for private health insurance sold to, or provided by large companies is usually the same for every employee with a family and is varied only for single persons. Age of employees, number of children and their ages, dual coverage of husband and wife when both are employed are all unknown factors in the base population. Utilization is reported by the identification number of the employee regardless of the family member involved.

The data on individuals in the population base and the individual's record of use of services could be designed into the system when it is created, but the insurance company needs only to determine rates that cover utilization costs. The insurance company has no need for analysis of these costs. If the insured company finds it desirable to know what it is paying for in some detail, the company must be willing to pay the costs of a more elaborate system of data collection.

Essentially, the same problems prevent the HMOs from producing utilization data. What data have been published both from insurance carriers and HMOs have been developed through special studies, designed to answer specific research problems.

In the future, utilization information for Medicare may also depend entirely on special studies or surveys. The Medicare system was established in 1966 with a statistical system that identified the insured individual and each service that was billed through the system. Medicare data will no longer be complete, however, with the growth of HMOs, the enactment of the law requiring first coverage of employed persons 65-70 by the employer, and the prospect of a possible voucher system.

Professional Association Data

Three major professional associations, the American Medical Association (AMA), the American Dental Association (ADA), and the American Nurses Association (ANA), have data bases relating to characteristics of their membership and/or of the profession they represent. The AMA maintains two data bases: the Physician Masterfile and the Socioeconomic Characteristics of Medical Practice. The Physician Masterfile contains information about all physicians, including non-AMA members, such as medical school attended and dates, year graduated, residency, board certification, licensure data, membership in professional societies, specialty (including geriatrics), and professional activities. The Socioeconomic Characteristics of Medical Practice file, published annually, contains information on the practice characteristics of a sample of active nonfederal office and hospital-based physicians drawn from the Masterfile, for example, patient care activities by specialty, professional expenses, fee schedules, and number of hours per week devoted to patient care.

The ADA conducts a similar membership survey. Its survey, however, contains information only on members of the ADA. This survey includes basic demographic, biographical, and practice characteristics of its members, such as schools attended and dates, year of graduation from dental school, location and type of practice (generalist or specialist), number of hours of practice per week. In addition, the ADA conducts sample surveys of about 5 percent of its members and nonmembers on practice characteristics, which include types of procedures used, fees charged, and age of patients treated.

The ANA conducts an annual survey of its members, which includes demographic, educational, employment, and worksite data. The major clinical, teaching, or practice area is specified, as is the job title, the specialty, the type of education received, and employment status (full or part time), and whether the individual is employed as a nurse. Data on the place or field of employment are also collected and include hospital, nursing home, school, HMO, community or home, occupational, and office nurse. No information on salaries is kept in this data base.

These association files provide little data related to services available for the elderly. The AMA Masterfile identifies physicians specializing in geriatrics; the ADA sample survey contains an item for age of patients; and the ANA specifies nursing home as a place of employment. Since the elderly use all types of services of physicians, dentists, and nurses, these files can provide information on the availability of professional services to the population of all ages, including the elderly, but not on the elderly as a group with special needs.

Summary

It should be remembered that the aforementioned data bases are not an exhaustive list. Rather they are illustrative of the variety of sources providing information, or working to provide information, to the public. Universities with gerontological centers are one example. In addition to the sources described there are a variety of private associations doing health-related research requiring that data bases be created for each roject. Quasi-academic settings are also sources of useful health policy data, for example, the Urban Institute, the Brookings Institution, and the Institute of Medicine.

11
Statistical Methodology for Health
Policy Analysis

INTRODUCTION

Previous chapters of this report have described the changing demographic profile of the U.S. population and the impact of the growing number of older Americans on demand for health, housing, and social services. They have also discussed the need for additional scientific research and policy-oriented analysis on patterns of aging and their consequences. Such investigations will require sophisticated use of existing statistical methodology and, in some cases, the development of new methods.

Although the importance of longitudinal information sometimes seems self-evident to investigators, the need for longitudinal studies and, conversely, the limitations of cross-sectional and retrospective investigations are not always apparent to decision makers and funding agencies. Thus, this chapter begins with a discussion of the rationale for longitudinal studies, followed by a discussion of problems in the design and analysis of longitudinal studies. A second major theme in this report is increased usage of existing studies and administrative information through linkage of data bases. The second section of this chapter is devoted to a discussion of some of the administrative, legal, and technical issues raised by attempts to link data bases. The third section of the chapter discusses methodological issues in a third area of fundamental importance in the study of aging, forecasting of the sizes and composition of populations, as well as population characteristics such as health status and needs for services. The final section of the chapter discusses a generic problem in policy analysis, the quantification and reporting of uncertainty.

LONGITUDINAL INFORMATION

The Rationale for Longitudinal Studies

Given the cost and complexity of developing longitudinal information for studies of any population and particularly the elderly, it is reasonable to ask why the data needed about the policy implications of an aging population cannot be obtained by simpler and less costly designs, especially cross-sectional studies. In subsequent paragraphs, we discuss two considerations that motivate longitudinal studies: (1) the need to study aging as a process and (2) the need to reduce bias and improve precision of estimates of net change in populations.

In many areas of investigation discussed in this report, the essential role of longitudinal data derives from the need to study aging and its consequences as processes, that is, complexes of states and events occurring over time (Rowe, 1977). Because these processes and the factors that determine their course are defined for individuals rather than population aggregates, they can be studied only by gathering data on individuals over time (Fienberg and Tanur, 1986). Examples of processes that must be understood in order to anticipate the needs of tomorrow's elderly include:

(1) The interaction between economic circumstances and health care utilization. One aspect of this interaction is the effect of acute and chronic illness on economic circumstances after retirement (Menefee, 1985), especially the spend-down to poverty that can occur during an extended illness. Another aspect is the effect of economic circumstances on patterns of health care utilization and the influence of different pathways on the economics of care (Meiners, 1985b).

(2) The dynamics of social networks involving elderly persons and the effects of social support on the subsequent physical and mental health of the elderly (Berkman, 1985).

(3) Patterns of morbidity and mortality in the elderly and the predictive significance of functional status, living conditions, and clinical risk factors (see Chapter 3).

By definition, these are questions about change—change in health or functional status, economic circumstances, or environment, and the resulting changes in utilization and costs of health, social, and housing services. More generally, the preceding chapters have identified a need for increased understanding of the transitions between states experienced by elderly persons and the dependence of these transitions on factors such as diseases, lifestyle habits, and changes in psychosocial supports. Only longitudinal data can provide the basic observations of change that are the objects of study.

Stochastic models can play an important role in the study of these phenomena. By formulating, fitting, and validating explicit models, statisticians can clarify multivariate relationships and refine projections of the health and service needs of tomorrow's elderly population. For example, models for relationships between health care costs and health care utilization can be used to examine the effects of changes in costs of medical services on future demand. Ideally a stochastic model for health care utilization and costs would also consider the role of personal health, personal economic resources, and other factors that influence health care needs. In practice, more complex models can be more difficult to validate and can also lead to more uncertain projections. Thus, stochastic modeling requires careful choices about model complexity.

Longitudinal data can be obtained either prospectively, by following individuals over time, or retrospectively, by obtaining historical information from study participants. Retrospective studies can play an important role in the study of aging, as evidenced by the ongoing NIA Survey of the Last Days of Life (National Research Council, 1986). They have important limitations, however, especially in studies of elderly persons. First, many subjective states or events cannot be reconstructed retrospectively. Similarly, physiologic measurements can be obtained only in prospective studies. Retrospective studies will also be affected by selective mortality. The absence of deceased persons from a retrospective study will produce an incomplete picture of the process under study. Finally, even objective states, such as changes in family composition or economic circumstances, are subject to inaccuracies of recall that can be especially severe in elderly persons. Thus, although retrospective studies can be of value, they do not provide a general methodologic alternative to longitudinal designs.

Longitudinal data are required for the study of gross flows and for the study of individual change and its determinants—studies that cannot be carried out with cross-sectional data. Although either longitudinal data or cross-sectional data can be used to provide data about net change in populations with age, several problems can be encountered in using cross-sectional data for this purpose. By net change, we mean the difference in age-specific distributions of population characteristics. As a specific example, we might wish to estimate the changes between ages 70 and 75 in percentages of persons who live in nursing homes and who need assistance with two or more activities of daily living. Using successive cross-sectional data, the percentage of 70-year-old residents requiring such assistance could be estimated at one year and the percentage of 75 residents requiring such assistance could be estimated 5 years later. This method could give a biased estimate of net change in that five-year period because of selective mortality.

In discussing mortality as a potential source of bias in cross-sectional data Rowe (1977) points out that whenever the variable under study is related to survival, a cross-sectional study can give biased estimates of age-related changes. In the study of changes in living conditions, for example, higher rates of mortality among individuals living in nursing homes would lead to underestimates of the age-specific rates of movement from independent living to nursing homes in cross-sectional data. Selective mortality can be viewed as a special kind of missing data problem; the effects of missing data on longitudinal analysis are discussed below.

Data from a single cross-sectional study could be used to make the comparison described above, which was based on sequential cross-sectional data. The percentage of 70-year-old residents needing assistance with two or more activities of daily living could be compared with the corresponding percentage of 75-year-old residents at the time of the study. Studying net change in this manner introduces the additional problem of cohort effects. Cohort effects in this instance would be differences between age-specific patterns of limitations in activies of daily living in cohorts born five years apart. The size of cohort effects can vary depending on the variable under study. One way to address the issue of cohort effects is to use successive cross-sectional data for the same cohort as described above. In view of these considerations, cross-sectional data can be used to obtain valid estimates of net change if the potential bias from selective mortality and cohort effects is small (Louis et al., 1986). Otherwise, longitudinal data are necessary for this purpose.

Finally, we note that longitudinal or repeated measures experiments are often designed to increase the precision of estimates of changes over time or between experimental conditions. Although this can also be a consideration in designing observational studies of aging, efficiency is typically a second-order consideration relative to considerations of informativeness and validity.

In summary, longitudinal designs are essential to the study of processes associated with aging and the factors determining their course because their focus on individuals encompasses patterns of improvement over time as well as decline. Cross-sectional data potentially can provide some information about net change in populations due to aging, but they can give biased, and possibly misleading, estimates when the variables under study are subject to cohort or selection effects.

Designing Longitudinal Studies

Although the design phase of longitudinal studies has received some attention in the statistical literature, most papers have addressed single issues in highly simplified settings. Several papers, for example, have investigated the relative efficiency of different repeated measures designs for estimating the average rate of change over time of a single measured variable. Schlesselman (1973) and Berry (1974) discussed the effect of duration and frequkency of measurement on the precision of estimated rates of change in measured physiologic variables such as pulmonary function or blood pressure measurements. For a review of this literature, see Cook and Ware (1983).

Design issues in more complex, possibly multipurpose, studies have not received the same attention, in part because the formulation of the issues is sensitive to the type of process and end point to be studied. One important class of questions involves the definition of units of study and end points. For example, longitudinal studies of family units require a longitudinal definition of the family. The Income Survey Development Program (David, 1983) defined households operationally by following members of the original household even when they moved away from the household group, but chose not to follow individuals entering the household after the original interview if they subsequently moved away. Each such decision creates opportunities and limitations in subsequent analysis. Similarly, when variables are measured repeatedly over time, special care is needed in developing measurement systems that are free of spurious temporal variation. This is easily appreciated in longitudinal studies of physiologic variables (Dawber, 1980) but equally important in the collection of questionnaire or interview data.

Every longitudinal study raises issues of this type, including the definition of study end points, the duration of study and frequency of measurement, the nature of the measurement system, the definition of study units, the nature of the sampling and follow-up plans, and many more such issues. We believe that resolution of these issues, critical to the success of complex studies, requires special consideration of the features of individual research settings. The panel urges that sponsors of longitudinal studies make provision in study staffing and timetables to allow for considerations of the special design problems posed by individual studies.

Designs and Their Implications for Longitudinal Data Analysis

In empirical applications, testing whether specific classes of stochastic process models describe the occurrence of events or the evolution of continuous variables is best facilitated by observing, in full, many realizations of the underlying process for all times in a wide time interval. Examples of such data are the work histories in the Seattle and Denver Income Maintenance Experiments (Tuma et al., 1979), the fertility histories in the Taichung IUD experiment (Freedman and Takeshita, 1969), and the job vacancy histories for ministers in Episcopalian churches in New England (White, 1970). In most substantive contexts, however, ascertaining the exact timing of each occurrence of an event for each individual is either impossible, economically infeasible, or both. Observations usually contain gaps and censoring relative to a continuously evolving process. Three examples of this situation are as follows:

(1) In the Framingham study (Dawber, 1980) of atherosclerotic disease, individuals were examined once every two years, at which times symptoms of illness, hospitalizations, or other events occurring between examinations were recorded (retrospective information). In addition, a physical examination, some blood studies, and other laboratory work (current information) were completed. One topic of considerable interest is the intraindividual dynamics of systolic blood pressure. This is a continuous-time and continuous-state process that can be modeled only using the biennial samples; i.e., measurements made at the examinations. Such data represent fragmentary information about the underlying process.

(2) In the Taeuber et al. (1968) residence history study, observations were taken retrospectively on current residence, first and second prior residence, and birthplace of individuals in particular

age cohorts. Analyses in which duration of residence is a dependent variable of interest must accommodate censoring on the right for current residence. Furthermore, characterizations of the pattern of adult residence histories is complicated by the fact that initial conditions are unknown for persons who have occupied more than three residences beyond, for example, age 18.

(3) The first Duke longitudinal study of aging was conducted on a sample of 271 male and female volunteers who were socioeconomically representative of elderly persons in the community of Durham, North Carolina. The mean age of the study population at the first test data was 71.3 years. At each of the 11 waves of the 21-year panel survey, a standard battery of physiological risk factors, serum cholesterol, diastolic blood pressure, and pulse pressure were ascertained from all persons still alive and in the study. Wechsler intelligence tests were also given to participants at each wave. In modeling the age-dependent risk factors that affect mortality in this elderly population (Manton and Woodbury, 1983b), the analyst must take account of the fact that (a) relative to continuously evolving processes, there are gaps in the data on the physiological risk factors—they are measured at most 11 distinct times in 21 years; (b) high rates of mortality selection and unequal follow-up times led to small sample sizes for studying risk factor changes at the most advanced ages, and (c) all variables are not necessarily recorded for all individuals present at a given survey, thereby yielding very intricate patterns of missing data within a survey and over time.

A feature of modeling with such fragmentary data is that algebraic characterizations of the data sets that can possibly be generated by given continuous-time models are frequently very difficult to obtain. However, these characterizations are, of necessity, the basis of tests for compatibility of the data with proposed classes of models. In addition, estimation of quantities such as rates of occurrence of events per individual at risk of the event at a given time is complicated by the fact that some of the occurrences are unobserved. This necessitates estimation of rates that have meaning within stochastic process models that are found to be compatible with the observed data.

Analytical Strategies

In the ideal but rather infrequent settings in which evolving processes are observed over a time interval, two quite disparate—in terms of historical roots—but nevertheless related modeling frameworks have been utilized to estimate rates of occurrence of events, changes in levels of continuous variables, and parameters associated with covariates that are viewed as the primary factors that influence outcomes. One of these modeling frameworks is a direct adaptation of the classical linear statistical models to longitudinal data, reviews of which are contained in Ware (1985) and Ware et al. (1988). Also see Geisser (1980) for pertinent review of the capabilities of longitudinal data analysis for making projections and predictions. An alternative framework, originating from diverse stochastic process specifications, is the multivariate counting process literature (see the review by Andersen and Borgan, 1984) and the multivariate Gaussian process and diffusion process literature (see in this regard Woodbury et al., 1979, Manton and Woodbury, 1983a). Applications of both the stochastic process framework and the linear models specifications in the context of labor economics and the sociology of work are discussed in detail in Heckman and Singer (1985).

For data with the types of limitations illustrated in the examples given above, a major research program remains to be carried out before longitudinal data analysis can be regarded as a mature subject. A commonly used analytical strategy proceeds according to the following basic steps:

(1)   When estimation of transition rates between a discrete set of states is the primary focus of the analysis, one begins with very simple, somewhat plausible classes of models as candidates to describe some portion of the observed data and within which the unobserved dynamics are well defined—for example, a time series of time-homogeneous Markov chains for which each separate model describes only unobserved dynamics between a pair of consecutive surveys in a multiwave panel design and fits the observed transitions.

(2)   Estimate and interpret the parameters of interest—for example, transition rates between discrete pairs of states—within the simplified models and then assess whether these models can, in fact, account for finer-grained detail such as the joint frequency of state occupancy at three or more consecutive surveys in a multiwave panel study.

(3)   Typically, the original proposed models—they are usually first-order Markovian across a wide range of subject matter contexts—that may adequately represent data based on pairs of consecutive surveys will not account for higher-order dependencies. Such

dependencies tend to be the rule rather than the exception in longitudinal microdata. We then look for structured residuals from the sample models to guide the selection of more realistic and interpretable specifications (see, e.g., Singer and Spilerman, 1976; Goodman, 1978; Duncan, 1981) for a discussion of this kind of strategy in a variety of sociology and economics investigations).

The repeated fitting of models and subsequent utilization of structured residuals to guide successively more realistic model selection is a strategy that, on the surface, seems to be very reasonable. However, the process frequently stagnates after only one or two stages because the possible explanations for given structured residuals are usually too extensive to be helpful by themselves. One really needs, in addition, specific subject matter theories translated into mathematics to guide the model selection process. Unfortunately, in most fields in which analysis of longitudinal microdata is of interest, the development of substantive theory is quite weak.

The potential danger of the foregoing strategy, even for the estimation of transition rates, is that parameter estimates may be biased simply as a result of model misspecifications. The biases, in turn, can lead to incorrect conclusions about relationships between events.

As the foregoing discussion suggests, considerable room remains for the development and assessment of stochastic models for temporal processes. Ideally these models will be based on mathematical constructs that represent the underlying biological, behavioral, or other processes in a meaningful way. Analytic methods should be applicable in settings in which data sets are unbalanced and incomplete. In some cases, it will be important to explicitly model the processes that lead to missing data. Although there are many successful examples of longtitudinal analysis, methodological approaches and applications are very diverse and approaches tend to differ in different applied settings. In particular, the econometric, sociometric, biometric, and human growth literatures contain extensive work on longitudinal methods, but communication among the groups of investigators is imperfect. One can hope that future methodological developments will lead toward more unified approches to model formulation and data analysis.

An important new development for exploring high-dimensional longitudinal data sets is the family of grade of membership (GOM) models developed by Woodbury et al. (1978), Woodbury and Manton (1982), and Manton et al. (1987). This modeling framework is well suited to studying the dynamics of highly heterogeneous elderly populations and has the added very desirable feature of breaking free of conventional regression structures when assessing the impact of covariates on outcome variables. The essential idea is to represent the individual histories in a vector stochastic process in terms of the evolution of degrees of similarity (or grades of membership) of individuals to ideal (or pure type) profiles. The profiles are characterized by combinations of levels on particular covariates that occur with high frequency. The profiles also need not be static. They may in fact be stochastic processes themselves, thereby leading to a representation of individual dynamics in terms of evolving degrees of similarity to special pure type processes. Although much further theoretical, empirical, and numerical computational development remains to be carried out before GOM can be considered to be a well understood and readily utilized framework, it has already shown sufficient promise in studies of health status dynamics and health care utilization in elderly populations to warrant much more sustained investigation.

A much neglected topic with both fragmentary and relatively complete longitudinal data is the recognition that choice-based sampling is a pervasive aspect of many data sets, and that it plays a particularly central role in program evaluation of almost every kind. For a very readable and insightful introduction to the analytical issues associated with choice-based samples and selection bias, see Heckman and Hotz (1987). This topic should be—but to date has not been—playing a major role in evaluations of health care systems for elderly populations. It is a research area critically in need of development.

Recommendation 11.1: Given the growing importance and complexity of longitudinal research, the panel recommends that federal agencies encourage methodological research on innovative approaches to study design and analysis, both through support of methodological work within their own technical groups and through funding of methodological research.

RECORD LINKAGE

The Rationale for Record Linkages

Many of the data requirements discussed in preceding chapters can be satisfied most economically by linking data from different sources. Linkages may be at the aggregate level or they may involve individual records from different data systems. Linkages of individual records may be accomplished either by exact matching or by statistical matching. In an exact match, the goal is to link records for the same individuals from two or more data systems; in a statistical match, the goal is to link records for individuals who are similar in important respects. Exact matching, if feasible, is a method to be adopted because fewer assumptions are needed to ensure the validity of analyses based on the linked data sets (U.S. Department of Commerce, 1980, Recommendation 1b, p.33).

Statistical purposes of record linkages include enhancement of survey data by adding data from administrative files, development of sampling frames for surveys and the evaluation of coverage and response errors in censuses and surveys. Important multipurpose statistical data systems have been developed by exact matching of records from different administrative files maintained by federal agencies.

Linkage of existing records as an alternative to direct data collection has become more appealing because of the development of sophisticated computerized record linkage techniques, based on models first proposed in the 1950s and 1960s (Newcombe et al., 1959; Fellegi and Sunter, 1969). Linkages are further facilitated by increasingly widespread use of Social Security numbers as identifiers (Jabine, 1985).

Examples of exact record linkages that have contributed or have the potential to contribute to our information base on the status of older Americans include:

- Linkage of administrative data on retirement benefits to survey data collected in the Social Security Administration's Retirement History Survey (Fox, 1979).
- Linkage of survey records from the Current Population Survey, the National Health Interview Survey, and the National Health and Nutrition Examination Survey to death records in the National Death Index (Patterson and Bilgrad, 1985).
- Linkage of survey records from the National Medical Care Utilization and Expenditures Survey to records in the Medicare and Medicaid administrative data files (Cox and Bonham, 1983).

- Linkage of Social Security Administration and Internal Revenue Service administrative records for a 1 percent longitudinal sample of persons in the Continuous Work History Sample System (Buckler and Smith, 1980).
- Linkage of administrative data from Social Security Administration and Internal Revenue Service files to Current Population Survey records in the 1973 Exact Match Study (Kilss and Scheuren, 1978).

This list of examples by no means exhausts the potential for innovative and efficient uses of record linkages to provide useful data on the status of older Americans.

Recommendation 11.2: The panel recommends that federal agencies support activities to facilitate linkage of federal data bases for policy analysis related to the aging population. Data bases considered for such linkages should include both surveys and files of administrative records, for example, Social Security retirement and Medicare benefit files. Agencies that maintain such data bases, including the Social Security Administration, the National Center for Health Statistics, the Census Bureau, and agencies that need improved information on the effects of an aging population, should seek opportunities to fund demonstration projects to explore additional methods for the creation and analysis of linked data bases. Whenever feasible these linkage studies should use exact matching of individual records rather than statistical matching.

Obstacles to the Use of Record Linkage Techniques

There are several factors that inhibit extensive use of record linkage techniques to meet data needs. These limiting factors are of two kinds: those that make it impossible or difficult to link records in the first place and those that inhibit full and effective use of the linked data files that are produced.

Obstacles to Performance of Record Linkages

Obstacles to carrying out record linkages include technical problems, resource constraints, legal constraints, and policy considerations. There has been considerable progress in the development of computerized record linkage techniques, but there are still many aspects for which significant technical improvements are possible. These aspects include, for example, the choice and standardization of matching variables, the choice of blocking strategies (blocking limits the comparison of records in two files to those that agree on certain variables that appear in both files) and the role of manual intervention in computerized systems. Matching errors inevitably occur in linked data files, so far relatively little has been done to assess these errors and to develop estimation and analysis techniques that take them into account. One source of error among the elderly is the often noted phenomenon of age misreporting (exaggeration) among those age 85 and over (Rosenwaike, 1968).

> **Recommendation 11.3:** The panel recommends that federal agencies support research aimed at the development of improved multipurpose computerized record linkage systems and better methods of estimation and analysis when matching errors are present.

Formats vary for recording identifiers such as names and addresses in statistical and administrative data files. Other potential matching variables, such as age (or date of birth), race, ethnic origin, and marital status are defined and categorized in various ways. These variations make record linkages more difficult and lead to matching errors.

> **Recommendation 11.4:** The panel recommends that federal agencies that maintain statistical or administrative data bases work together to encourage standardization of definitions and reporting formats for personal identifiers (the Social Security number is critically important) and personal characteristics likely to be used as matching variables.

Although in the long run some data requirements can be met more economically by linking existing records, it is often difficult to obtain the necessary resources. Substantial research and development efforts may be needed to explore feasibility and to adapt existing record linkage programs to make them suitable for a specific application. Understandably, agencies like the Social Security Administration and the Internal Revenue Service that maintain potentially useful administrative data systems do not consider the development of statistical data bases not directly related to their own programs to be a high-priority activity. Therefore most of the resources must come from potential users, some of whom may be reluctant to invest significant amounts in the development of data systems over which they will have relatively little control.

Statutes like the 1974 Privacy Act, the Census Bureau's Title 13, and the Tax Reform Act of 1976 restrict, in varying degrees, the disclosure of individually identifiable data by one agency to another. Nevertheless, interagency record linkages can usually be undertaken in ways that do not violate statutory prohibitions, provided the agencies controlling the record systems involved are sufficiently motivated to do the linkage. These statutory limitations may, however, be considered obstacles to record linkages in two senses. First, they provide a convenient argument against performing a particular record linkage for an agency that is not anxious to do it. Second, even when both agencies want to do the linkage, the time required for development and approval of suitable arrangements can often substantially delay completion of a project, adversely affecting the utility of results.

> **Recommendation 11.5:** The panel recommends that heads of appropriate federal agencies take the initiative to seek methods of overcoming legal and policy obstacles to cost-effective use of existing information through linkages that are clearly beneficial to the public and ethical, and that they seek legislative remedies if necessary.

Policy considerations are probably the primary obstacle to successful record linkage undertakings. Both statistical and administrative agencies are concerned that public cooperation with their requirements or requests for information may be adversely affected if it becomes widely known that they are allowing such information to be linked with the records of other agencies. The Privacy Act, however, requires that people who supply information be informed of any plans to disclose such information in individually identifiable form. Agencies vary considerably in the amount of detail they provide in their Privacy Act notification statements: this is an ethical dilemma that has received some recent attention (Scheuren, 1985).

These concerns are by no means groundless. Computers, data banks, and record linkages are, rightly or wrongly, viewed with concern or suspicion by a substantial segment of the public. Even those agencies that have mandatory authority to collect information depend heavily on voluntary cooperation to obtain the data they need. Any widely publicized report of deception or other improper behavior on their part, whether accurate or not, could have serious repercussions. A recent example is the controversy that erupted in Sweden, early in 1986, concerning privacy aspects of Project Metropolitan, a sociological record linkage study designed to follow, over a 20-year period, all 10-year-olds who lived in Stockholm in 1963. Nonresponse in Sweden's monthly labor force survey has more than doubled in recent months, apparently as a result of the public debate about Project Metropolitan (Dalenius, 1986).

Obstacles to Dissemination and Use of Record Linkage Results

For record linkages that are undertaken despite the obstacles just described, the benefits derived depend on how widely and in how much detail the resulting data are disseminated to potential users. Publicly collected data are disseminated in two forms: aggregate statistics and microdata files. The latter contain individual records from which explicit identifiers, such as name and address, have been removed (microdata files that can be released without restriction are called public-use files). Statistical agencies have been releasing public-use microdata files for about 30 years, and the widespread availability of these files has benefited society by increasing the amount and relevance of quantitative information available for collective decision making.

Agencies that release data for statistical purposes must attempt, whether or not the data are derived from linked records, to avoid disclosing information in a form that makes it possible to identify specific individuals and thereby learn more about them. In other words, they must avoid statistical disclosure. Methods used to limit the risk of statistical disclosure resulting from release of microdata files include elimination of some geographic and other detail, replacement of exact amounts with class intervals, and deliberate introduction of error.

In practice, zero risk of disclosure is unattainable (Cox et al., 1985). The development of powerful computerized record linkage techniques has increased the likelihood of success by someone who, for whatever reason, might deliberately try to identify one or more persons from a public-use microdata file. Recent research by Paass (1985) suggests that deliberate introduction of random errors into records does not provide effective protection but does hamper the intended uses of the data. More recently, Duncan and Lambert (1986) introduced a "disclosure limiting" (DL) approach that provides a framework for measuring the extent of statistical disclosure if specific aggregated statistical data are released. They have demonstrated that certain ad hoc disclosure control policies commonly used by statistical agencies are special cases of the DL approach. Although microdata would fit into the context of the DL approach, use of DL with this type of data has not yet been explored.

Concerns about statistical disclosure risks have led to curtailment of the amount of information released in the form of microdata files. The extreme case is that of the Continuous Work History Sample (CWHS). Since shortly after the passage of the Tax Reform Act of 1976, no CWHS microdata files have been released because of findings by the Internal Revenue Service that there is a nonzero risk of disclosing individual tax return information. Prior to that time, CWHS microdata files were widely used by researchers inside and outside government to study relationships between earnings and benefits, internal migration, labor mobility, industry, mortality, and other topics. Plans had been developed to enhance the CWHS with data on mortality, retirement benefits, and Medicare benefits, thus creating a longitudinal data file of great potential value for research on policy issues related to the health of the aging population. The CWHS is a 1 percent sample of all persons who have ever been issued Social Security numbers and therefore provides virtually complete coverage of older persons. It is large enough (as of 1984 it included about 250,000 persons age 65 and over who receive Social Security benefits) to support analyses for subgroups of the elderly defined geographically or in other ways. The amount of longitudinal data is unmatched by other data sources.

Unfortunately, when releases of CWHS microdata files were terminated in 1976, the plans for content expansion through linkage with other files had to be terminated. Limited efforts along these lines are presently under way as a collaborative project of the Statistics of Income Division of the Internal Revenue Service and the Office of Research, Statistics, and Internal Policy of the Social Security Administration, with funding from the National Cancer Institute. The panel recognizes the Continuous Work History Sample as a potentially valuable data base for research on policy issues relating to health, Medicare benefits, disability, and mortality of the aging population. It supports current efforts of the Internal Revenue Service and the Social Security Administration to enhance the system and resume limited dissemination of microdata files.

Recommendation 11.6: The panel recommends that the Social Security Administration and the Internal Revenue

Service conduct a comprehensive review of the Continuous Work History Sample system, with a view to resuming broader release of its products under user agreements. If necessary, legislative authority should be sought. Federal agencies with information requirements that can be met by enhancing the CWHS system are urged to provide budgetary support.

Releases of public-use microdata files from the decennial censuses, the Current Population Survey, and other sources, some of which include linked administrative records, have continued. However, many users, including other federal agencies, have said that their uses of the files are hampered by the content restrictions that the releasing agencies impose in order to maintain the risk of statistical disclosure at what they consider to be an acceptably low level.

Recommendation 11.7:   The panel recommends that federal statistical agencies develop procedures for making microdata files more readily available to users, including both other federal agencies and nongovernment researchers. Technical procedures, such as curtailment of file content and the deliberate introduction of error, cannot reduce the risk of statistical disclosure to zero; therefore, other methods of protecting the confidentiality of data subjects should be explored. Such methods include user agreements with penalties for violation and legal remedies for data subjects harmed by disclosure.

PROJECTIONS FOR AN AGING POPULATION

The future needs of the aged population depend on its size, composition, morbidity and mortality rates, educational and economic status, housing and living arrangements, and also on the unpredictable changes in the incidence and treatment of illness. The aged population has a dynamic nature in both size and composition because of new entrants (people who reach the age of 65) and those who die. During the next 20 years, the new entrants into the aged population, persons now ages 45-64, represent a cohort that differs from the cohort now ages 65-84 in educational, marital, income, health, and other characteristics (Myers, 1985). The informed evaluation of issues pertaining to policy decision making for this aging population requires forecasts for the years 2000 and beyond that will account for the forthcoming demographic and societal developments.

The Bureau of the Census issues basic population projections for the future composition of the national population by age, race, and sex as well as by state and region. These projections also provide a basis for others, such as those concerning educational status, marital status, household structure, and labor force status—all of which are single-factor projections. The other general type of forecast, which is discussed later in the chapter, is interactive models that can account for the effect of factors on each other.

A noteworthy limitation of these Census Bureau projections is their lack of regularity. The most recent set was released in final form in May 1984, and the previous set in 1977. The periods covered by these projections have also tended to vary widely, with more recent sets extending farther into the future (Myers, 1985).

Recommendation 11.8: The panel recommends that a basic set of projections be prepared by the Bureau of the Census every 10 years based on the decennial census and covering all characteristics included in the past—age, race, sex, marital status, living arrangements, and educational attainment. Ethnicity, migration, and greater geographic detail are also needed. A shorter-term projection should be prepared five years after release of the projection based on decennial census data.

The Bureau of the Census has used methodology similar to that of the Social Security Administration to produce future population estimates for its program. An important contribution made by Social Security is to forecast mortality. These estimates take into account trends in cause-specific mortality by age and sex but not race. Their construction also involves judgmental procedures with potentially arbitrary assumptions about the patterns of change in mortality rates over time. This issue merits attention for assessments of health status when more extensive consideration of the biological process is useful, particularly in the development of morbidity and disability forecasts. Cooperation with the Health Care Financing Administration and the National Center for Health Statistics in these efforts is essential. The Health Care Financing Administration has produced forecasts of national health expenditures and types of expenditures to the year 1990 on the basis of Social Security Projections (Freeland and Schendler, 1983). Also, the National Center for Health Statistics has reported on projections of various aspects of health services utilization and health care expenditures for the year 2003 (National Center for Health Statistics, 1983b).

As noted previously, important factors in many projections concerning population size, composition, and health status are the levels of age-specific mortality rates in the future. The mortality rates provided through Social Security account for age, sex, major disease category, and judgments about patterns of variation over time. However, they are not differentiated by race.

> **Recommendation 11.9:** The panel recommends that race be used in addition to age and sex in mortality rates by disease and in forecasting the size and health status of the population.

Dissemination of data from projections has tended to be mainly in the form of published tables showing particular age and characteristic information for some specific points in time. For example, in 1979 the Census Bureau projected marital status for the period 1979-1995 focusing on 10-year age intervals for 1985, 1990, and 1995. In addition, the input schedules for the change components and related assumptions may not be presented in published reports in adequate detail. One way of overcoming these limitations of published tables is to release information in tape form or through interactive computer systems. These would enable users to have their own capability of preparing their own alternative projections.

> **Recommendation 11.10:** The panel recommends that agencies release projections and underlying information in tape form as well as in published tables and that documentation of basic assumptions in the projections accompany the tape and the published tables.

There are several sources of uncertainty which influence the accuracy of projections for the elderly population. Data quality at older ages is one important consideration; potential problem areas include age misstatement, underenumeration, and inaccurate reporting of characteristics, as well as nonresponse at the characteristic and entire person levels. An additional well-known source of variability in surveys is sampling variability. Its role for older ages can be substantial when the sample size for older age groups is very small. Another important source of uncertainty for projections is sensitivity to assumptions such as those concerning the magnitude and pattern of change of mortality rates. The previously stated considerations merit attention for projections concerning an aging population because the rates of transition between relevant states at older ages are often much greater than those at younger ages. For example, the mortality rate for males ages 45-49 was 546.1 per 100,000 in 1982, but nearly 20 times greater at ages 80-84. Higher transition rates among the elderly also apply to morbidity, hospitalization, and other experiences. As a consequence of these issues, the level of error experienced in estimation are greater at older ages, so care needs to be given to managing such uncertainty and describing its implications in order to avoid potentially misleading findings and subsequently misguided policy (Myers, 1985).

> **Recommendation 11.11:** The panel recommends that agencies describe the nature of uncertainty for projections. The basis of estimates of uncertainty should also be documented in terms of underlying sources such as those for data quality, sampling variability, and sensitivity to assumptions.

Many of the factors that are of interest for an aging population interact with one another. One way to account for such interactions is through global models that attempt to integrate different submodels or modules into a common projection framework. Such models can have either an aggregate economic-demographic structure or a microsimulation structure for a created population of individuals. Two noteworthy examples of the former type with specific features in their designs for studies of the elderly are the Macroeconomic-Demographic Model (National Institute on Aging, 1984a) and the Demographic-Economic Model of the Elderly (Olsen et al., 1981). The Demographic-Economic Model of the Elderly (DECO) is part of a larger model developed by Data Resources, Inc. It provided 25-year projections of the economic implications of an aging population.

The Macroeconomic-Demographic Model (MDM) was initiated under the President's Commission on Pension Policy and has been further developed by the National Institute on Aging. It is a long-term model intended to assess how the changing age structure of the population will affect the income level of the elderly as well as productivity, consumption, savings, and investment. The model treats all population factors exogenously within the comprehensive, integrated model of long-term economic growth and labor force supply and demand. These, in turn, are related to major features of national pension systems and transfer programs. Research is under way for the development of modules to assess the demand for health insurance and services and another on health expenditures. These modules would appear to require further detail on health status. The model could benefit from the development of more endogenous modules for the demographic component with respect to family formation and dissolution, fertility, health status, and mortality.

Microsimulation models involve Monte Carlo procedures that can apply different patterns of transitions to the individuals in a sample population. When adequate estimation of their parameters is feasible, they can enable evaluation of factors that can affect changes in distributions of population characteristics such as health status or health services utilization. Examples of useful microsimulation models include POPSIM (a product of the Research Triangle Institute), DYNASIM (prepared by the Urban Institute: Wertheimer and Zedlewski, 1980); and a preliminary research model designed by the Duke University Center for Demographic Studies to examine future health status (Myers et al., 1977).

Another consideration in the development of forecasting models is the incorporation of more biomedical information. A recent effort in this direction is described in Manton (1985). Incidence and prevalence of cancer morbidity by age group to age 90 and over are projected to the year 2000 under assumptions of a changing population structure and one fixed from 1977. Projections of lung cancer deaths in the year 2000 under both assumptions were made. An interesting feature of these forecasts is their linkage to stochastic compartment modeling techniques for the estimation of health state transitions for persons subject to specific diseases. Multiple sources of data are used to deal with age cohort differences in risk, changes in risk over the life span, individual differences in risk, and both independent and dependent competing risk assumptions about interactions among diseases (Myers, 1985).

As discussed here, developments are needed that would lead to more sophisticated modeling of the components of population, particularly the mortality component that so affects the projections of the aged population. In this regard, integrated efforts are necessary to forecast health status, functional limitations, and support systems available for older persons (Manton, 1984). Not only can these forecasts have utility for probing important policy issues related to health care expenditures and welfare programs, but they also can be informative for improved mortality forecasts in general population projections. The NIA recognized the importance of forecasting methodology and recently issued a Request for Applications on the methodology of forecasting active and disabled life expectancy.

Recommendation 11.12: The panel recommends that a study to evaluate theoretical, methodological, and data requirements for forecasting the characteristics of the aging population be undertaken. This would include theoretical and practical considerations for evaluating the sensitivity of forecasts to underlying assumptions.

The Bureau of the Census and the National Institute on Aging would be appropriate agencies to fund this study.

QUANTIFYING UNCERTAINTY

In a paper prepared for the panel, Stoto (1985) discussed the problem of quantifying the uncertainty associated with projections or other data summaries produced in policy-oriented analysis. These difficulties have two principal sources: (1) the need for assumptions that cannot be verified and (2) the use of data bases that arise from poorly defined stochastic models.

The inability to verify critical assumptions about the adequacy of the stochastic model beyond the range of the available data is intrinsic to projection. Stoto discusses several approaches to the characterization of uncertainty in projection. One important methodology is sensitivity analysis, the evaluation of the changes induced in a projection by changes in key assumptions or parameters. Sensitivity analysis is sometimes summarized through the reporting of high, middle, and low projections. Regrettably, many policy analyses do not include a discussion of the sensitivity of key findings to unverifiable assumptions.

Similarly, many policy analyses involve the collection and integration of data from a variety of sources. The analysis of such data sets requires special methods or higher-level models that link the information from different sources. This problem has received considerable attention in the statistical and social-scientific literature, under the rubrics *risk assessment* (DuMouchel and Harris, 1983) and *meta-analysis* (Glass, 1976). Many research workers are concerned with methodology for combining data from different sources (see, for example, Hedges and Olkin, 1985; Wolf, 1986; Gupta and Wilton, 1987).

Speaking more generally, much of statistical methodology is

based on the paradigm of a well-defined experiment or sampling plan. Critical information required for decision making, however, is often not of this type but is rather more diffuse and less clearly structured. The analysis of such information poses a challenge to statisticians and other quantitative scientists, as has been recognized by many and has led to considerable research on policy analysis, as well as the formation of new professional groups such as the Society for Decision Analysis. The panel believes that this line of research is very important not only to policy analysis on the consequences of an aging population, but also to policy analysis in many other areas of importance to this country. We believe also that further advances in understanding of methods for conducting and reporting policy oriented analyses are critically needed.

Recommendation 11.13: The panel recommends that federal agencies relying on quantitative analysis to guide policy encourage and support research on methods for conducting and reporting policy analyses, especially methods for quantifying the uncertainty of projections and data summaries.

References

Aday, L.A., and Andersen, R.
  1975   *Development of Indices of Access to Medical Care.* Ann Arbor, Mich.: Health Administration Press.
Adler, G.S.
  1982   Evaluation Options for Medicaid. Technical Appendix: Review of HCFA Data Sources. Urban Systems Research and Engineering, Inc., Cambridge, Mass. and Systemetrics, Inc., Lexington, Mass.
Aloia, J.F., Cohn, S.H., Ostuni, J.A., Cane, R., and Ellis, K.
  1978   Prevention of involutional bone loss by exercise. *Annals of Internal Medicine* 89:356-358.
Andersen, P.K., and Borgan, O.
  1984   Counting Process Models for Life History Data: A Review. Research Report 84/2, Statistical Research Unit, University of Copenhagen.
Andersen, R.M., McCutcheon, A., Aday, L.A., Chiu, G.Y., and Bell, R.
  1983   Exploring dimensions of access to medical care. *Health Service Research* 18(1):49-74.
Anderson, W.F.
  1966   The prevention of illness in the elderly: The Rutherglen experiment in medicine in old age. *Proceedings of a Conference Held at the Royal College of Physicians.* London: Pitman.
Andrews, F., and Withey, S.R.
  1976   *Social Indicators of Well-being: Americans' Perceptions of Life Quality.* New York: Plenum Press.
Bergner, M.
  1985   Measurement of health status. *Medical Care* 23(5).
Berkman, L.F.
  1985   Maintenance of Health—Prevention of Disease: A Psychological Perspective. Paper prepared for Panel on Statistics for an Aging Population, Committee on National Statistics, National Research Council.

259

Berkman, L.F., and Breslow, L.
1983   *Health and Ways of Living: The Alameda County Study.* New York: Oxford University Press.

Berry, G.
1974   Longitudinal observations: Their usefulness and limitations with special reference to the forced expiratory volume. *Bulletin de Physiopathologie Respiratoire* 10:129-145.

Besdine, R.W.
1982   The data base of geriatric medicine. Pp. 1-15 in J.W. Rowe and R.W. Besdine, eds., *Health and Disease in Old Age.* Boston: Little, Brown.
1983   The educational utility of comprehensive functional assessment in the elderly. *Journal of the American Geriatric Society* 31:651-656.
1984   Functional Assessment in the Elderly: Relationships Between Function and Diagnosis. Paper presented at the Fifth Annual Symposium on the Elderly and Their Health, Department of Epidemiology and Preventive Medicine, School of Medicine, University of Maryland.

Bharadwaj, L.K., and Wilkening, E.A.
1977   The prediction of perceived well-being. *Social Indicators Research* 4:421-439.
1980   Life domain predictors of satisfaction with personal efficacy. *Human Relations* 33:165-181.

Blanchet, M.
1986   Advances in Preventive Medicine. Paper presented at the Colloquium on Aging with Limited Health Resources, Economic Council of Canada, Winnipeg, Manitoba.

Blendon, R.J.
1986   Health policy choices for the 1990s. *Issues in Science and Technology* 2(4):65-73.

Branch, L.G., and Jette, A.M.
1982   A prospective study of long-term care institutionalization among the aged. *American Journal of Public Health* 72:1373-1379.
1984   Personal health practice and mortality among the elderly. *American Journal of Public Health* 74:1126-1129.

Brody, E.
1981   Women in the middle. *The Gerontologist* 21(5):471-480.

Brody, J.A.
1987   The best of times and the worst of times: Aging and dependency in the 21st century. Pp. 3-21 in S.F. Spicker, S.R. Ingman, and I.R. Lawson, eds., *Ethical Dimensions of Geriatric Care.* Boston: D. Reidel Publishing Co.

Brook, R.H., and Lohr, K.N.
1985   Efficacy, effectiveness, variations and quality: Boundary-crossing research. *Medical Care* 23(5):710-722.

Buckler, W., and Smith, C.
1980   The Continuous Work History Sample (CWHS): Description and contents. Pp. 165-174 in *Economic and Demographic Statistics.* Washington, D.C.: U.S. Department of Health and Human Services, Social Security Administration.

Busse, E.W., and Maddox, G.L.
   1985   *Longitudinal Study of Normal Aging, 1955-1980. An Overview of History, Design, and Findings.* New York: Springer Publishing Company.
Campbell, A., Converse, P.E., and Rodgers, W.L.
   1976   *The Quality of American Life.* New York: Russell Sage Foundation.
Cook, N., and Ware, J.H.
   1983   Design and analysis methods for longitudinal research. *Annual Review of Public Health* 4:1-23.
Cornoni-Huntley, J., Brock, D.B., Ostfeld, A.M., Taylor, J.O., and Wallace, R.B., eds.
   1986   Established Populations for Epidemiologic Studies of the Elderly: Resource Data Book. National Institute of Aging. NIH Publication #86-2443. Washington, D.C.: National Institutes of Health.
Council of Professional Associations on Federal Statistics (COPAFS).
   1986   *News from COPAFS.* No. 50. October. Council of Professional Associations on Federal Statistics, Washington, D.C.
Cox, B., and Bonham, G.
   1983   Sources and solutions for missing data in the NMCUES. Pp. 444-449 in *Proceedings of the Section of Survey Research Methods.* Washington, D.C.: American Statistical Association.
Cox, L., Johnson, B., McDonald, S., Nelson, D., and Vazquez, V.
   1985   Confidentiality issues at the Census Bureau. Pp. 199-218 in *Proceedings, First Annual Research Conference.* Washington, D.C.: U.S. Bureau of the Census.
Cross, P.S., and Gurland, B.J.
   1986   The Epidemiology of Dementing Disorders. Contract report prepared for the Office of Technology Assessment, U.S. Congress. Washington, D.C.: U.S. Government Printing Office.
Crozier, D.
   1985   DataWatch. *Health Affairs* 4(spring):114-128.
Dalenius, T.
   1986   The 1986 Invasion of Privacy Debate in Sweden. Unpublished report, Brown University.
David, M.
   1983   *Technical, Conceptual, and Administrative Lessons of the Income Survey Development Program.* New York: Social Science Research Council.
Davis, K.
   1985   Access to health care: A matter of fairness. Pp. 45-47 in *Health Care: How to Improve It and Pay for It.* Washington, D.C.: Center for National Policy.
Davis, K., and Rowland, D.
   1986   *Medicare Policy: New Directions for Health and Long-Term Care.* Baltimore: Johns Hopkins University Press.
Dawber, T.
   1980   *The Framingham Study: The Epidemiology of Atherosclerotic Heart Disease.* Cambridge, Mass.: Harvard University Press.
Donabedian, A.
   1980   *Explorations in Quality Assessment and Monitoring, Volume I: The Definition of Quality and Approaches to Its Assessment.* Ann Arbor, Mich.: Health Administration Press.

Doty, P.
1986　　Family care of the elderly: The role of public policy. *Milbank Memorial Fund Quarterly* 64(1):34-75.

Doty, P., Liu, K., and Weiner, J.
1985　　Special report: An overview of long-term care. *Health Care Financing Review* 6(3):69-78.

DuMouchel, W.H., and Harris, J.E.
1983　　Bayes methods for combining the results of cancer studies in humans and other species. *Journal of the American Statistical Association* 78:293-315.

Duncan, G.T., and Lambert, D.
1986　　Disclosure-limited data dissemination. *Journal of the American Statistical Association* 81:10-18.

Duncan, O.D.
1981　　Two faces of panel analysis. In S. Leinhardt, ed., *Sociological Methodology, 1981.* San Francisco: Jossey-Bass.

Elder, Charles D., and Coble, Roger W.
1984　　Agenda building and the politics of aging. *Policy Studies Journal,* 13:115-129.

Etheredge, Lynn
1987　　*Redesigning Medicare: A Comparison of Benefit and Financing Reform Proposals.* Prepared by the Consolidated Consulting Group for the National Health Policy Forum. Washington, D.C.: National Health Policy Forum.

Feder, J.M., and Scanlon, W.M.
1980　　Regulating the bed supply in nursing homes. *Milbank Memorial Fund Quarterly* 58(1):34-88.

Feldman, J.J.
1983　　Work ability of the aged under conditions of improving mortality. *Milbank Memorial Fund Quarterly* 61:430-444.

Fellegi, I., and Sunter, A.
1969　　A theory of record linkage. *Journal of the American Statistical Association* 64:1183-1210.

Fienberg, S.E., and Tanur, J.M.
1986　　The design and analysis of longitudinal surveys: Controversies and issues of cost and continuity. Pp. 60-93 in R. Boruch and R. Pearson, eds., *Survey Research Designs: Towards a Better Understanding of Their Costs and Benefits.* Lecture Notes in Statistics, Volume 38. New York: Springer-Verlag.

Fienberg, S.E., Loftus, E.F., and Tanur, J.M.
1985　　Cognitive aspects of health surveys for public information and policy. *Milbank Memorial Fund Quarterly/Health and Society* 63(3).

Fillenbaum, Gerda G.
1984　　*The Wellbeing of the Elderly: Approaches to Multidimensional Assessment.* Geneva: World Health Organization.

Filner, B., and Williams, T.F.
1981　　Health promotion for the elderly: Reducing functional dependence. Pp. 187-204 in A.R. Somers, and D.R. Fabian, eds., *The Geriatric Imperative: An Introduction to Gerontology and Clinical Geriatrics.* New York: Appleton-Century-Croft.

Fox, A.
1979   Pre-retirement earnings patterns: Evidence from the Retirement
          History Study. Pp. 265-270 in *Proceedings of the Social Statistics
          Section.* Washington, D.C.: American Statistical Association.
Franklin, J.L., Solovitz, B., and Simmons, J.
1984   Quality of Life of the Chronically Mentally Ill. Paper presented
          November 11-16, 1984 at the annual meeting of the American Public
          Health Association, Anaheim, Calif.
Franks, P., Lee, P.R., and Fullarton, J.E.
1983   Lifetime Fitness and Exercise for Older People. A background
          paper prepared for the Administration on Aging, U.S. Depart-
          ment of Health and Human Services. Aging Health Policy Center,
          University of California, San Francisco.
Freedman, R., and Takeshita, J.Y.
1969   *Family Planning in Taiwan.* Princeton, N.J.: Princeton University
          Press.
Freeland, M.S., and Schendler, C.E.
1983   National health expenditure growth in the 1980s: An aging pop-
          ulation, new technologies, and increasing competition. *Health Care
          Financing Review* 4(3):1-58.
Fries, James F.
1980   Aging, natural death, and the compression of morbidity. *New
          England Journal of Medicine* 303(3):130-135.
1983   The compression of morbidity. *Milbank Memorial Fund Quarterly*
          61:397-419.
Fullerton, H.N., Jr.
1980   The 1995 labor force: A first look. *Monthly Labor Review* 103(12):11-
          21.
Garfinkel, S.A., and Corder, L.
1984   *Supplemental Health Insurance Coverage Among Aged Medicare Beneficia-
          ries.* Series B. Descriptive Report 5. Washington, D.C.: Health
          Care Financing Administration, Office of Research and Demonstra-
          tions.
Gastil, R.
1978   Social indicators and quality of life. *Public Administration Review*
          30:596-601.
Geisser, S.
1980   Growth curve analysis. Pp. 89-115 in P.R. Krishnaiah, ed., *Handbook
          of Statistics*, Vol. 1. New York: North-Holland Publishing Company.
George, L., and Bearon, L.
1980   *Quality of Life in Older Persons: Meaning and Measurement.* New York:
          Human Sciences Press.
German, P.S.
1981   Measuring functional disability in the older population. *American
          Journal of Publc Health* 71(11):1197-1199.
German, P.S., Klein, L.E., McPhee, S.J., and Smith, C.R.
1982   Knowledge of and compliance with drug regimens in the elderly.
          Journal of the American Geriatric Society 30:568-571.
Gilson, B.S., Michnich, M.E., Thompson, R.S., and Friedlander, L.
1984   Physician Effectiveness in Preventive Care Project. Investigation

supported by the U.S. Department of Health and Human Services, Public Health Service, National Center for Health Services Research. Grant No. 1 R18 HS 04387-01.

Ginsburg, P.B., and Hackbarth, G.M.
    1986   Alternative delivery systems and Medicare. *Health Affairs* (spring):6-22.

Glass, G.V.
    1976   Primary, secondary and meta-analysis of research. *Educational Researcher* 5:3-8.

Goldschmidt-Clermont, Luisella
    1982   Product Related Evaluation of Unpaid Household Work: A Challenge for Time Use Studies. Unpublished paper. Institute de Sociologie, Universite Libre de Bruxelles.

Goodman, L.A.
    1978   *Analyzing Qualitative/Categorical Data.* Cambridge, Mass.: Abt Books.

Gordon, Nancy M., for the U.S. Congressional Budget Office
    1986   Statement to Subcommittee on Health and the Environment, Committee on Energy and Commerce, U.S. House of Representatives. March 26.

Gornick, M., Greenberg, J.N., Eggers, P.W., and Dobson, A.
    1985   Twenty years of Medicare and Medicaid: Covered populations, use of benefits, and program expenditures. *Health Care Financing Review Annual Supplement*:13-59.

Greenfield, S., Cretin, S., Worthman, L.G., Dorey, F., Solomon, N., and Goldberg, G.
    1981   Comparison of a criteria map to a criteria list in quality of care assessment for patients with chest pain: The relation of each to outcome. *Medical Care* 19(3):255-272.

Gruenberg, Ernest M.
    1977   The failures of success. *Milbank Memorial Fund Quarterly/Health and Society* 55(1):3-24.

Gupta, S., and Wilton, P.C.
    1987   Combination of forecasts: An extension. *Management Science* 3:352-372.

Hall, M.J.
    1983   Mental illness and the elderly. Pp. 483-505 in R.J. Vogel and H.C. Palmer, eds., *Long-Term Care, Perspectives from Research and Demonstrations.* Washington, D.C.: Health Care Financing Administration.

Health Care Financing Administration
    1985a   *Medicare Program Statistics.* Baltimore, Md.: Bureau of Data Management and Strategy.
    1985b   Project to Redesign Information Systems Management (PRISM). Office of Information Resources Management, Bureau of Data Management and Strategy. October.

Heckman, J., and Hotz, V.J.
    1987   Do we need experimental data to evaluate the impact of manpower training or earnings? *Evaluation Review* 11(4):395-427.

Heckman, J., and Singer, B.
    1985   *Longitudinal Analysis of Labor Market Data,* New York: Cambridge University Press.

Hedges, L.V., and Olkin, I.
1985   *Statistical Methods for Meta-Analysis.* New York: Academic Press.

Herzog, A.R., Rodgers, W.L., and Woodworth, J.
1982   Subjective Well-being Among Different Age Groups. Research Report Series, Survey Research Center, University of Michigan.

Hodgson, T.A., and Meiners, M.
1982   Cost-of-illness methodology: A guide to current practices and procedures. *Milbank Memorial Fund Quarterly* 60(3):429-462.

Horn, S.D., and Horn, R.A.
1986   The computerized severity index: A new tool for case mix management. *Proceedings of the 19th Annual Hawaii International Conference on Systems Science.*

Hu, T., and Sandifer, F.H.
1981   Synthesis and Cost of Illness Methodology. National Center for Health Services Research Contract No. 233-79-3010. Public Services Laboratory, Georgetown University.

Institute of Medicine
1986   *Improving the Quality of Care in Nursing Homes.* Committee on Nursing Home Regulations, Institute of Medicine. Washington, D. C.: National Academy Press.

Interagency Statistical Committee on Long-Term Care of Elderly
1980   Data coverage of the functionally limited elderly: Report of the Interagency Statistical Committee on Long-Term Care of Elderly. *Statistical Reporter* 80(10):281-316.

Inui, T.S., and Carter, W.B.
1985   Problems and prospects for health services research on provider-patient communication. *Medical Care* 23(5).

Jabine, T.
1985   Properties of the social security number relevant to its use in record linkages. Pp. 213-226 in B. Kilss and W. Alvey, eds., *Record Linkage Techniques 1985.* Washington, D.C.: U.S. Department of the Treasury, Internal Revenue Service.

Jajich, C.L., Ostfeld, A.M., and Freeman, D.H., Jr.
1984   Smoking and coronary heart disease mortality in the elderly. *Journal of the American Medical Association* 252:2831-2834.

Kane, R.A., and Kane, R.L.
1981   *Assessing the Elderly: A Practical Guide to Measurement.* Lexington, Mass.: Lexington Books.

Kane, R.L., Kane, R.A., and Arnold, S.B.
1985   Prevention and the elderly: Risk factors. *Health Services Research* 19 (February, Part II):945-1005.

Kane, R.L., Solomon, D., Beck, J., Keeler, E., and Kane, R.
1980   Geriatric manpower in the United States. *New England Journal of Medicine.* 302(24):1327-1332.

Kane, R.L., Solomon, D., Beck, J., Keeler, E., and Kane, R.
1981   *Geriatrics in the United States. Manpower Projections and Training Considerations.* Lexington, Mass.: Lexington Books.

Katz, S., Branch, L.G., Branson, M.H., Papsidero, J.A., Beck, J.C., and Greer, D.S.
1983   Active life expectancy. *New England Journal of Medicine* 309:1218-1224.

Katz, S., Greer, D.S., Beck, J.C., Branch, L.G., and Spector, W.D.
  1985   Active life expectancy. In *America's Aging: Health in an Older Society*.
          Committee on an Aging Society, Institute of Medicine and National
          Research Council. Washington, D.C.: National Academy Press.
Katzman, R.
  1985   Aging and age-dependent disease: Cognition and dementia. Pp.
          129-152 in *America's Aging: Health in an Older Society*. Committee
          on an Aging Society, Institute of Medicine and National Research
          Council. Washington, D.C.: National Academy Press.
Kessner, D.M., Kalk, C.E., and Singer, J.
  1973   Assessing health quality—The case for tracers. *New England Journal
          of Medicine* 288(January):189-194.
Kilss, B., and Scheuren, F.
  1978   The 1973 CPS-IRS-SSA Exact Match Study. *Social Security Bulletin*
          41(10):14-22.
Kleinman, J.C., Gold, M., and Makuc, D.
  1981   Use of ambulatory medical care by the poor: Another look at
          equity. *Medical Care* 19:1011-1029.
Koizumi, A.
  1982   Toward a healthy life in the twenty-first century. Chapter 6 in
          *Population Aging in Japan: Problems and Policy Issues in the Twenty-first
          Century*. Chiyodaku, Tokyo, Japan: Nihon University.
Kovar, M.G.
  1986   Expenditures for the medical care of elderly people living in the
          community in 1980. *The Milbank Quarterly* 64(1):100-132.
Kramer, F., ed.
  1988   *From Quality Control to Quality Improvement in AFDC and Medi-
          caid.* Committee on National Statistics, National Research Council.
          Washington, D.C.: National Academy Press.
Kramer, Morton
  1980   The rising pandemic of mental disorders and associated chronic
          diseases and disorders. *Acta Psychiatrica Scandinavica Supplement*
          285(62):382-396.
  1981   The Increasing Prevalence of Mental Disorders: Implications for
          the Future. Paper presented at the National Conference on the
          Elderly Deinstitutionalized Patient in the Community, Arlington,
          Va.
Lakatta, E.G.
  1985   Health, disease, and cardiovascular aging. Pp. 73-104 in *America's
          Aging: Health in an Older Society*. Committee on an Aging Society,
          Institute of Medicine and National Research Council. Washington,
          D.C.: National Academy Press.
Lawton, M.P.
  1977   *Planning and Managing Housing for the Elderly.* New York: Wiley.
Lee, P.R.
  1985   Health promotion and disease prevention for children and the el-
          derly. *Health Services Research* 19 (February, Part II):783-792.
Lessler, J.T., and Sirken, M.G.
  1985   Laboratory-based research on the cognitive aspects of survey meth-
          odology: The goals and methods of the National Center for Health

Statistics study. *Milbank Memorial Fund Quarterly/Health and Society* 63(3).

Lichtenstein, P., Sneen, M., and Yaffe, R.
No date Medicare Automated Data Retrieval System (MADRS). Health Care Financing Administration, Baltimore, Md.

Liu, K., Manton, K.G., and Liu, B.M.
1985 Home care expenses for the disabled elderly. *Health Care Financing Review* 7(2):51-58.

Longino, C.F., Jr., Beggar, J.C., Flynn, C.B., and Wiseman, R.F.
1984 The Retirement Migration Project. A Final Report to the National Institute on Aging. Center for Social Research in Aging. University of Miami, Coral Gables, Florida.

Louis, T.A., Robins, J., Dockery, D.W., Spiro, A. III, and Ware, J.H.
1986 Explaining discrepancies between longitudinal and cross-sectional models. *Journal of Chronic Disease* 39(10):836-839.

Lowy, L.
1983 Social policies and programs for the elderly as mechanisms of prevention. Pp. 7-21 in S. Simson, L.B. Wilson, J. Hermalin, and R. Hess, eds., *Aging and Prevention: New Approaches for Preventing Health and Mental Health Problems in Older Adults.* New York: Haworth Press.

Lubitz, J., and Prihoda, R.
1984 Use and costs of Medicare services in the last 2 years of life. *Health Care Financing Review* 5:117-131.

Mangen, D.J., and Peterson, W.A., eds.
1982 *Research Instruments in Social Gerontology.* Volume 1, Clinical. Minneapolis: University of Minnesota.

Manton, K.G.
1982 Changing concepts of morbidity and mortality in the elderly population. *Milbank Memorial Fund Quarterly/Health and Society* 60(2):183-244.
1984 Methods and issues in the projections of population health status. *World Health Statistics Quarterly* 37:294-305.
1985 Models for Forecasting the Health Status of the Elderly. Paper presented at the Workshop on Forecasting Life and Active Life Expectancy, National Institute on Aging, Bethesda, Md.
1986a Measurement of Health and Disease: A Transitional Perspective. Paper prepared for Panel on Statistics for an Aging Population, Committee on National Statistics, National Research Council.
1986b The Linkage of Health Status Changes and Workability. Paper presented at the Workshop on Prevention as a Way to Improve Work Capacity in Older People, Brookings Institution, Washington, D.C.

Manton, K., and Soldo, B.
1985 Long Range Planning for the Elderly: An Integrated Policy Perspective. Paper prepared for the U.S. Senate Special Committee on Aging.

Manton, K.G., Stallard, E., Woodbury, M.A., Tolley, H.D., and Yashin, A.
1987 Grade of membership techniques for studying complex event history processes with unobserved covariates. In C. Clogg, ed., *Sociological Methodology, 1987.* San Francisco: Jossey-Bass.

Manton, K.G., and Woodbury, M.A.
    1983a   A mathematical model of the physiological dynamics of aging and correlated mortality selection: I. Theoretical development and critiques. *Journal of Gerontology* 38(4):398-405.
    1983b   A mathematical model of the physiological dynamics of aging and correlated mortality selection: II. Application to the Duke Longitudinal Study. *Journal of Gerontology* 38(4):406-413.

Maslow, A.H.
    1954   *Motivation and Personality.* New York: Harper and Row.

Mathematica Policy Research, Inc.
    1986   Evaluation of the National Long-Term Care Demonstration: Final Report Executive Summary. Prepared by George J. Carcagno and others for HCFA, ADA, ASPE, Department of Health and Human Services. Princeton, N.J.: Mathematica Policy Research, Inc.

Meiners, M.R.
    1985a   Long term care insurance. *Generations* (summer)39-42.
    1985b   Data Requirements for Long-term Care Insurance. Paper prepared for the Panel on Statistics for an Aging Population, Committee on National Statistics, National Research Council.

Menefee, J.A.
    1985   Economic Data and the Analysis of Health-related Issues of the Elderly. Paper prepared for the Committee on National Statistics, Panel on Statistics for an Aging Population, National Research Council.

Minaker, K.L., and Rowe, J.W.
    1985   Health and disease among the oldest old: A clinical perspective. *Milbank Memorial Fund Quarterly* 63:324-349.

Mohr, K.H.
    1985   *Peer Review Organizations (PROs): Quality Assurance in Medicare.* Paper prepared for Office of Technology Assessment, U.S. Congress. Washington, D.C.: U.S. Government Printing Office.

Morgan, J.N., and Smith, J.D.
    1969   Measures of economic well-offness and their correlates. *American Economic Review* 59:912-926.

Murnaghan, J.H., ed.
    1976   *Long-Term Care Data.* Report of the Conference on Long-Term Health Care Data. Philadelphia, Pa.: J.B. Lippincott Company.

Myers, George C.
    1985   Research for Tomorrow's Elderly. Paper prepared for the Panel on Statistics for an Aging Population, Committee on National Statistics, National Research Council.

Myers, G.C., Pitts, A.M., Hillson, R., and Stallard, E.
    1977   A microsimulation model for health status projections. Pp. 694-700 in *Proceedings of the Social Statistics Section of the American Statistical Association, Part II.* Washington, D.C.: American Statistical Association.

Najman, J.M., and Levine, S.
    1981   Evaluating the impact of medical care and technologies on the quality of life: A review and critique. *Social Science and Medicine* 15F(June-September):107-115.

National Center for Health Statistics
1981   Characteristics of Nursing Home Residents, Health Status, and Care Received: National Nursing Home Survey, United States, May-December 1977. *Vital and Health Statistics.* Series 13, No. 51. DHHS Publication No. (PHS) 81-1712, Washington, D.C.: U.S. Department of Health and Human Services.

1983a   *Americans Needing Help to Function at Home.* Public Health Service Advance Data No. 92, DHHS Pub. No. 83-1250. Washington, D.C.: U.S. Department of Health and Human Services.

1983b   Changing mortality patterns: Health services utilization and health care expenditures, United States, 1978-2003. *Vital and Health Statistics,* Series 3, No. 23. Washington, D.C.: U.S. Department of Health and Human Services.

1984a   NCHS Monthly Vital Statistics Report. Vol. 32, No. 10, Supplement (2). February 17. Public Health Service. Washington, D.C.: U.S. Department of Health and Human Services.

1984b   *Patterns of Ambulatory Care in Internal Medicine: The National Ambulatory Medical Care Survey.* United States, January 1980-December 1981. Series 13, No. 80. DHHS Publication No. (PHS)84-1741. Hyattsville, Md: National Center for Health Statistics.

1985a   *National Health Interview Survey,* Health Promotion and Disease Prevention Supplement, Form HIS-1(SB). Hyattsville, Md: National Center for Health Statistics.

1985b   *1984 Summary: National Hospital Discharge Survey.* DHHS Publication No. (PHS)85-1250. Hyattsville, Md.: National Center for Health Statistics.

1985c   Public Use Data Tape Documentation. Dental, Ages 1-74. Tape Number 4235 of National Health and Nutrition Examination Survey, 1971-1975.

1986a   Advance report of final mortality statistics, 1984. *Monthly Vital Statistics Report* 35:6, Supplement 2. DHHS (PHS) 86-11.20. Public Health Service. Washington, D.C.: U.S. Department of Health and Human Services.

1986b   Current estimates from the National Health Interview Survey, United States, 1985. P. 114, Table 71 in *Vital and Health Statistics,* Series 10, No. 160. DHHS Pub. No. (PHS) 86-1588. Hyattsville, Md.: National Center for Health Statistics.

1986c   *Health United States, 1985.* DHHS Pub. No. PHS 86-1232. Public Health Service. Washington, DC: U.S. Government Printing Office.

1987a   Design Alternatives for Integrating the National Medical Expenditure Survey with the National Health Interview Survey. *Vital and Health Statistics.* Series 2, No. 101. DHHS Publication No. (PHS) 87-1375, Washington, D.C.: U.S. Department of Health and Human Services.

1987b   1985 Summary National Ambulatory Medical Care Survey. T. McLemore and J. Delozier. Advance Data from Vital and Health Statistics, No. 128. DHHS Publication No. (PHS) 87-1250. National Center for Health Statistics.

National Health Policy Forum
1985   *Addressing Medical Practice Variations: A Challenge for PROs and Private*

Review Agencies. Issue Brief No. 409. Washington, D.C.: George Washington University.

1986 *The Quality of Health Care: The Peer Review Process and Beyond.* Issue Brief, No. 456:II. Washington, D.C.: George Washington University.

National Institute on Aging

1984a *The National Institute on Aging Macroeconomic-Demographic Model.* NIH Publication No. 84-2492. Washington, D.C.: National Institutes of Health.

1984b *Report on Education and Training in Geriatrics and Gerontology.* National Institute on Aging. February.

1985 Implementation Plan, Health Research Extension Act of 1985. Part G, Section 8. Study of Personnel for Health Needs of the Elderly. National Institute on Aging.

National Research Council

1984 *Rural America in Passage: Statistics for Policy.* D.M. Gilford, C.L. Nelson, and L. Ingram, eds. Washington, D.C.: National Academy Press.

1986 Inventory of data sets related to the health of the elderly. Prepared by the Panel on Statistics for an Aging Population, Committee on National Statistics. Pp. 241-266 in *Statistical Policy for an Aging America.* Joint Hearing of the Subcommittee on Energy, Nuclear Proliferation, and Government Processes and the Subcommittee on Governmental Affairs. 99th Congress, 2nd Session. Washington, D.C.: U.S. Government Printing Office.

Newcombe, H., Kennedy, J., Axford, S., and James, A.

1959 Automatic linkage of vital records. *Science* 130:954-959.

Office of Technology Assessment

1985a *Medicare's Prospective Payment System: Strategies for Evaluating Cost, Quality, and Medical Technology.* OTA-H-262. Washington, D.C.: U.S. Government Printing Office.

1985b *Technology and Aging in America.* OTA-BA-264. Washington, D.C.: U.S. Government Printing Office.

1987 *Losing a Million Minds: Confronting the Tragedy of Alzheimer's Disease and Other Dementias.* OTA-BA-323. Washington, D.C.: U.S. Government Printing Office.

Olson, L., Caton, C., and Duffy, M.

1981 *The Elderly and the Future Economy.* Lexington, Mass.: Lexington Books.

Paass, G.

1985 Disclosure Risk and Disclosure Avoidance for Microdata. Paper presented at meeting of the International Association for Social Service Information and Technology, Amsterdam.

Patterson, J., and Bilgrad, R.

1985 The National Death Index experience: 1981-1985. Pp. 245-254 in *Record Linkage Techniques—1985.* Internal Revenue Service. Washington, D.C.: U.S. Department of the Treasury.

Peskin, J.

1983 The Value of Household Work in the 1980s. Paper presented at the American Statistical Association meeting, Toronto, Ont.

President's Commission for the Study of Ethical Problems in Medicine and Biomedical and Behavioral Research
1983   *Securing Access to Health Care: The Ethical Implications of Differences in Availability of Health Services*, Vol. 1. Washington, D.C.: U.S. Government Printing Office.
President's Reorganization Project for the Federal Statistical System
1981   Improving the federal statistical system: Issues and options. *Statistical Reporter* 81:5.
Rabin, D.L.
1985   Waxing of the gray, waning of the green. Pp. 28-56 in *America's Aging: Health in an Older Society*. Committee on an Aging Society, Institute of Medicine and National Research Council. Washington, D.C.: National Academy Press.
Radloff, L.S.
1977   The CES-D scale: A self-report depression scale for research in the general population. *Applied Psychological Measurement* 1(3):385-401.
Rice, Dorothy P.
1985   The health care needs of the elderly. Pp. 41-66 in Charlene Harrington, Robert J. Newcomer, Carroll L. Estes, and associates, eds., *Public Policy Issues in Long-Term Care*. Beverly Hills, Calif.: Sage Publications.
1986   The medical care system: Past trends and future projections. *The New York Medical Quarterly* 6:39-70.
Rice, D.P., and Feldman, J.J.
1983   Living longer in the U.S.: Demographic change in health needs of the elderly. *Milbank Memorial Fund Quarterly/Health and Society* 61(3):362-396.
Rice, D.P., Hodgson, T.A., and Kopstein, A.N.
1985   The economic costs of illness: A replication and update. *Health Care Financing Review* 7(1):61-80.
Rice, T., and McCall, N.
1985   The extent of ownership and the characteristics of Medicare supplemental policies. *Inquiry* 22(2):188-200.
Riley, G., Lubitz, J., Prihoda, R., and Stevenson, M.A.
1985   *Changes in the Distribution of Medical Expenditures Among Aged Enrollees 1969 to 1982*. Working Paper Series No. 85-12. Washington, D.C.: Health Care Financing Administration.
Roos, N.P., Shapiro, E., and Havens, B.
1986   Aging With Limited Resources: What Should We Really Be Worried About? Paper presented at Colloquium on Aging with Limited Health Resources, Economic Council of Canada, Winnipeg, Manitoba.
Rosenwaike, Ira
1968   On measuring the extreme aged in the population. *Journal of the American Statistical Association* 63:29-40.
1985   A demographic portrait of the oldest old. *Milbank Memorial Fund Quarterly Health and Society* 63(2).
Rosow, I., and Breslau, N.
1966   A Guttman health scale for the aged. *Journal of Gerontology* 21:556-559.

Rowe, J.W.
1977   Clinical research on aging: Strategies and directions. *New England Journal of Medicine* 297:1332-1336.
1983   Isolated systolic hypertension in the elderly. *New England Journal of Medicine* 309:1246-1247.
1985   Health care of the elderly. *New England Journal of Medicine* 312(13): 827-835.

Russell, L.B.
1987   Evaluating Preventive Care: Report on a Workshop. Brookings Institution, Washington, D.C.

Rutstein, D.D., Berenberg, W., Chalmers, T.C., Child, C.G. III, Fishman, A.P., and Perrin, E.B.
1976   Measuring the quality of medical care: A clinical method. *New England Journal of Medicine* 294(11):582-588.

Sanazaro, P.J.
1985   A survey of patient satisfaction, knowledge, and compliance. *Western Journal of Medicine* (142):703-705.

Sawyer, D., Ruther, M., Pagan-Berlucchi, A., and Muse, D.
1983   *The Medicare Medicaid Data Book.* Health Care Financing Administration Publication 03156. Baltimore, Md.: U.S. Department of Health and Human Services.

Scheuren, F.
1985   Methodological issues in linkage of multiple data bases. Paper prepared for the Panel on Statistics for an Aging Population, Committee on National Statistics, National Research Council.

Schlesselman, J.J.
1973   Planning a longitudinal study. I. Sample size determination. II. Frequency of measurement and study duration. *Journal of Chronic Diseases.* 26:553-560, 561-570.

Schneider, Edward L. and Brody, Jacob A.
1983   Aging, natural death, and the compression of morbidity: Another view. *New England Journal of Medicine* 309(14):854-856.

Serow, William J., and Sly, David F.
1985   The Demography of Current and Future Aging Cohorts. Paper presented at the Symposium on a Social and Built Environment in an Aging Society, Committee on an Aging Society, Institute of Medicine and National Research Council.

Shanas, E.
1982   *National Survey of the Aged.* DHHS Pub. No. (OHDS)83-2045. Washington, D.C.: U.S. Department of Health and Human Services.

Shanas, E., and Maddox, G.L.
1985   Health, health resources, and the utilization of care. In R.H. Binstock, and E. Shanas, eds., *Handbook of Aging and the Social Sciences,* 2nd edition. New York: Van Nostrand Reinhold Company.

Shapiro, S.
1984   Provider-based surveys of health care use from the National Center for Health Statistics: An appraisal of their scope and content. *Health Services Research* 19(April):133-137.

1986   Are elders underserved? *Generations* 10(spring):14-17.

Shapiro, S., Skinner, E.A., Kramer, M., Steinwachs, D.M., and Regier, D.A.
1985   Measuring need for mental health services in a general population. *Medical Care* 23(9):1033-1043.

Siegel, J., and Davidson, M.
1984   Demographic and Socioeconomic Aspects of Aging in the United States. *Current Population Reports*. Special Studies Series P-23, No. 138. Washington, D.C.: U.S. Department of Commerce.

Singer, B., and Spilerman, S.
1976   Some methodological issues in the analysis of longitudinal surveys. *Annals of Economic and Social Measurement* 5(4):447-474.

Smith, E.L., and Reddan, W.
1976   Physical activity—A modality for bone accretion in the aged. *American Journal of Roentgenology Radiation Therapy and Nuclear Medicine* 126:1297.

Smith, E.L., Jr., Reddan, W., and Smith, P.E.
1981   Physical activity and calcium modalities for bone mineral increase in aged women. *Medical Science Sports Exercise* 13:60-64.

Soldo, B.J., and Manton, K.G.
1985   Changes in the health status and service needs of the oldest old: Current patterns and future trends. *Milbank Memorial Fund Quarterly/Health and Society* 63(spring):286-319.

Somers, Anne R.
1987   Insurance for long-term care: Some definitions, problems, and guidelines for action. *New England Journal of Medicine* 317(1):23-29.

Stoiber, M.S.
1979   A view from the administration. P. 167 in *Proceedings of the Public Health Conference on Records and Statistics: The People's Health: Facts, Figures, and the Future.* DHEW Publication (PHS) 79-1214. Hyattsville, Md.: National Center for Health Statistics.

Stoto, M.A.
1985   Statistics for an Aging Population: Dealing with Uncertainty. Paper prepared for the Panel on Statistics for an Aging Population, Committee on National Statistics, National Research Council.

Strehler, B.L.
1975   Implications of aging for society. *Proceedings of the Federation of American Societies for Experimental Biology* 34:5-8.

Taeuber, Cynthia
1983   America in transition: An aging society. *Current Population Reports*, Special Studies Series P-23, No. 128. Bureau of the Census. Washington, D.C.: U.S. Department of Commerce.

Taeuber, K.E., Chiazze, L., Jr., and Haenszel, W.
1968   *Migration in the United States: Analysis of Residence Histories.* Public Health Monograph No. 77. Edited and issued by Public Health Reports. Washington, D.C.: U.S. Department of Health, Education, and Welfare.

Tarlov, A.R.
1986   HMO growth and physicians. *Health Affairs* (spring):23-35.

Thier, Samuel O.
1986   Health policy: The critical issues. *Issues in Science and Technology* II(3):3-6.

Torrey, Barbara B.
1985   Sharing increasing costs on declining income: The visible dilemma of the invisible aged. *Milbank Memorial Fund Quarterly Health and Society.* 63(2):377-394.

Torrey, Barbara B., Kinsella, Kevin, and Taeuber, Cynthia M.
1987   An aging world. *International Population Report*, No. 78. Bureau of the Census. Washington, D.C.: U.S. Department of Commerce.

Tuma, N., Hannan, M. and Groeneveld, L.
1979   Dynamic analysis of event histories. *American Journal of Sociology* 84:820-854.

U.S. Congress
1984   Public Law 98-551, Sec. 1706. Centers for Research and Demonstration of Health Promotion and Disease Prevention.
1985   Study of personnel for health needs of the elderly. Health Research Extension Act of 1985, Public Law 99-158, Sec. 8.

U.S. Congress, Senate
1976   Committee on Post Office and Civil Service. Committee Print No. 2, Title 13, United States Code—Census. 94th Congress, 2nd Session. December 31. Washington, D.C.: U.S. Government Printing Office.
1986a   *Aging America: Trends and Projections, 1985-86 Edition.* Prepared by the U.S. Senate Special Committee on Aging in conjunction with the American Association of Retired Persons, the Federal Council on the Aging, and the Administration on Aging. Washington, D.C.: U.S. Department of Health and Human Services.
1986b   The current state of the coordination of the U.S. statistical policy. Statement of James T. Bonnen in *The Quality of the Nation's Economic Statistics.* Senate Document 99-865:302-320. Hearings before the Joint Economic Committee. Washington, D.C.: U.S. Government Printing Office.

U.S. Congressional Budget Office
1984   *Veterans Administration Health Care: Planning for Future Years.* Washington, D.C.: U.S. Government Printing Office.

U.S. Department of Commerce
1980   *Report on Exact and Statistical Matching Techniques.* Statistical Policy Working Paper 5. Office of Federal Statistical Policy and Standards. Washington, D.C.: U.S. Department of Commerce.

U.S. Department of Health, Education, and Welfare
1979   *Healthy People: The Surgeon General's Report on Health Promotion and Disease Prevention, 1979.* DHEW Publication No. (PHS) 79-55071. Washington, D.C.: Department of Health, Education, and Welfare.

U.S. Department of Health and Human Services
1980a   *Promoting Health/Preventing Disease: Objectives for the Nation.* Washington, D.C.: U.S. Public Health Service, U.S. Department of Health and Human Services.
1980b   *Report of the National Committee on Vital and Health Statistics. Long-Term Health Care, Minimum Data Set.* DHHS Pub. No. (PHS)80-1158. Hyattsville, Md.: Office of Health Research, Statistics, and Technology, National Center for Health Statistics.
1980c   Uniform Hospital Discharge Data, Report of the National Committee on Vital and Health Statistics. DHHS Pub. No. (PHS)80-1157.

Hyattsville, Md.: Office of Health Research, Statistics, and Technology, National Center for Health Statistics.

1983   Promoting health/preventing disease: Public health service implementation plans for attaining the objectives for the nation. *Public Health Reports* (supplement to September-October 1983 issue). Washington, D.C.: Public Health Service, Office of the Assistant Secretary for Health, Office of Disease Prevention and Health Promotion.

1984   U.S. Preventive Services Task Force Fact Sheet, July. Public Health Service, Office of Disease Prevention and Health Promotion. Washington, D.C.

1985   *The Public and High Blood Pressure: Six-Year Follow-up Survey of Public Knowledge and Reported Behavior.* NIH Publication No. 85-2118. Washington, D.C.: National Institutes of Health.

1986a   *Fifth report to the President and Congress on the Status of Health Personnel in the United States.* Executive Summary. Introduction, Summary, and Highlights. Bureau of Health Professions. Washington, D.C.: U.S. Department of Health and Human Services.

1986b   *Issues Regarding the Aged* and accompanying letter from Harold Loe, Director, NIDR, to T. Franklin Williams, April 15, 1986 for Agenda of Summit Meeting on Aging-Related Statistics. Washington, D.C.: National Institutes of Health.

1986c   *Research Activities* No. 82. National Center for Health Services Research and Health Care Technology.

1987   *Personnel for Health Needs of the Elderly Through Year 2020.* Executive Summary: Bethesda, Md: National Institute on Aging.

U.S. Office of Management and Budget
1985   *Federal Statistics: A Special Report on the Statistical Programs and Activities of the United States Government - Fiscal Year 1986.* Office of Information and Regulatory Affairs. Washington, D.C.: U.S. Government Printing Office.

Valvona, J., and Sloan, F.
1985   DataWatch: Rising rates of surgery among the elderly. *Health Affairs* 4.

Van Nostrand, J.F.
1985a   Data Gaps in Long-Term Care Policy Analysis. Paper presented at the annual meeting of the Gerontological Society of America, New Orleans, La.

1985b   Data Needs for Policy Analysis of Long-Term Care. Paper presented at the annual meeting of the American Public Health Association, Washington, D.C.

Veterans Administration
1984   *Caring for the Older Veteran.* Washington, D.C.: Veterans Administration.

Vinokur, A., Cannell, C.F., Eraker, S.A., Juster, F.T., Lepkowski, J.M., and Mathiowetz, N.
1983   *Cost-Effectiveness of Pharmaceuticals Report Series.* Report 6: The Role of Survey Research in the Assessment of Health and Quality-of-Life Outcomes of Pharmaceutical Interventions. Ann Arbor, Mich.: Institute for Social Research/University of Michigan.

Waldo, D., and Lazenby, H.
1984   Demographic characteristics and health care use and expenditures by the aged in the U.S.: 1977-1984. *Health Care Financing Review* 6(1):1-29.
Waldo, D.R., Levitt, K.R., and Lazenby, H.
1986   National Health Expenditures, 1985. *Health Care Financing Review* 8(1):1-21.
Wallman, Katherine K.
1985   Coordination of Federal Statistics Related to the Elderly. Paper prepared for the Panel on Statistics for an Aging Population, Committee on National Statistics, National Research Council.
Ward, G.W.
1984   The national high blood pressure education program. Pp. 93-113 in *Marketing Health Behavior: Principles, Techniques, and Applications.* New York: Plenum Press.
Ware, J.H.
1985   Linear models for the analysis of longitudinal studies. *The American Statistician* 39:95-101.
Ware, J.H., Lipsitz, S., and Speizer, F.E.
1988   Issues in the analysis of repeated categorical response. *Statistics in Medicine* 7(1):95-107.
Wertheimer, R.F., and Zedlewski, S.R.
1980   *The Aging of America: A Portrait of the Elderly in 1990.* Washington, D.C.: Urban Institute.
White, H.C.
1970   *Chains of Opportunity.* Cambridge, Mass.: Harvard University Press.
Wilkins, R., and Adams, O.
1983   *Healthfulness of Life.* Montreal: The Institute for Research on Public Policy.
Williams, M.E., Hadler, N.M., and Earp, J.A.L.
1982   Manual ability as a marker of dependency in geriatric women. *Journal of Chronic Diseases* 35:115-122.
Wilson, L.A., Larson, I.R., and Brass, W.
1962   Multiple disorders in the elderly: A clinical and statistical study. *Lancet* 2:841-843.
Wingard, D.L., Berkman, L.F., and Brand, R.J.
1982   A multivariate analysis of health-related practices: A nine-year mortality follow-up of the Alameda County Study. *American Journal of Epidemiology* 116:765-775.
Wolf, F.M.
1986   *Meta-Analysis: Quantitative Methods for Research Synthesis.* Beverly Hills, Calif.: Sage Publications.
Woodbury, M.A., Clive, J., and Garson, A.
1978   Mathematical typology: A grade of membership technique for obtaining disease definition. *Computers in Biomedical Research* 11:277-298.
Woodbury, M.A., and Manton, K.G.
1982   A new procedure for analysis of medical classification. *Methods of Information in Medicine.* 21:210-220.

Woodbury, M.A., Manton, K.G., and Stallard, E.
  1979   Longitudinal analysis of the dynamics and risks of coronary heart disease in the Framingham Study. *Biometrics* 35:575-585.
World Health Organization
  1948   Proceedings and Final Act of the International Health Conference New York 19 June - 20 July 1946. Official Records of the World Health Organization. United Nations WHO Interim Committee, Geneva, Switzerland.
  1984   The Uses of Epidemiology in the Study of the Elderly: Report for a WHO Scientific Group on the Epidemiology of Aging. Technical Report Series 706, Geneva, Switzerland.
  1986   *The Effectiveness of Health Promotion for the Elderly.* Report of a WHO Advisory Group. Hamilton, Ont.: World Health Organization.
Young, D.A.
  1985   Government payers for health care. Pp. 554-564 in *Assessing Medical Technologies.* Institute of Medicine. Washington, D.C.: National Academy Press.

Appendix A
Background Papers

Health and Related Issues

Measurement of Health and Disease: A Transitional Perspective
Kenneth G. Manton, Center for Demographic Studies, Duke University

Economic Data and the Analysis of Health Related Issues of the Elderly
John A. Menefee, Wyatt Company

Maintenance of Health — Prevention of Disease: A Psychosocial Perspective
Lisa Berkman, Department of Epidemiology, Yale School of Medicine

Statistical Methodology for Policy Analysis

Health Indicators for an Aging Population
Laurence G. Branch, Department of Social Medicine and Public Health, Harvard Medical School; *Julius B. Richmond*, Harvard University Division of Health Policy, Harvard Medical School; *David E. Rogers*, The Robert Wood Johnson Foundation; *Ronald W. Wilson*, Division of Epidemiology and Health Promotion, National Center for Health Statistics; *Mary M.E. Adams*, Francis A. Countway Library of Medicine, Harvard Medical School

Methodologic Issues in Linkage of Multiple Data Bases
    Fritz Scheuren, Internal Revenue Service

Statistics for an Aging Population: Dealing With Uncertainty
    Michael A. Stoto, John F. Kennedy School of Government, Harvard University

Improvement of Data Resources for Policy Analysis on Aging

Coordination of Federal Statistics Related to the Elderly
    Katherine Wallman, Council of Professional Associations on Federal Statistics

Research for Tomorrow's Elderly
    George C. Myers, Center for Demographic Studies, Duke University

Data Needs for Policy Analysis of Long-Term Care
    Joan Van Nostrand, National Center for Health Statistics

Lessons From Longitudinal Surveys
    Clifford Patrick, Social Security Administration

Data Requirements for Long-Term Care Insurance
    Mark Meiners, National Center for Health Services Research

State Data Issues for an Aging Population
    Charlene Harrington and Leslie Grant, Aging Health Policy Center, University of California, San Francisco

Appendix B
Effects of Budgetary Constraints on Federal Statistical Programs

The federal statistical agencies have responded to the changing fiscal environment of the last decade with a variety of broad policy changes and specific program adjustments. In many cases, these changes have been made hastily, without adequate consideration of their short- and long-term consequences, and thus have not supported the development of well-informed public policy.

In an era when the economy and the society are changing rapidly, these changes may be reducing the quantity and quality of vital information available to the public and private sectors for setting policy. With respect to the tasks of this panel, it is clear that the demographics of the elderly population are changing rapidly, that technology in health care and delivery systems is developing at a swift pace, and that the challenges posed to the medical community derive from the fact that the health care needs of an elderly population are not strictly defined by medical problems, but involve the social structures, home systems, and economic capacities of people as well.

As concerns statistics on the elderly, federal statistical agencies have been making changes to programs and policies in recent years that involve one or more of the following: (1) changing the focus from policy-oriented statistical programs to those that support the administrative aspects of government; (2) reducing the periodicity (or frequency of data collection) of major surveys; (3) reducing the coverage of surveys, through deletion of specific subpopulations from the universes of interest or through reduction of sample size; (4) reducing data quality, in the areas of data collection, data processing, and data dissemination; (5) reducing the timeliness of data dissemination, both in terms of hard-copy reports and of public-use data files; and (6) postponing or eliminating the regular review of data needs in developing areas, usually in the interest of protecting core programs within agencies.

Specific examples of the types of adjustments cited above are considered in the following sections, which examine the programs of the specific agencies that most directly affect the information bases available for supporting policy development in aging.

BUREAU OF THE CENSUS

There have been important effects of budget reductions on the products associated with the decennial census program. Unidentifiable effects on data quality may have been caused by the large-scale release of temporary employees hired to process the 1980 census early in the 1980s. A reduction-in-force of the permanent staff, conducted at the same time, caused major dislocation within the Bureau, both reducing total staff resources and relocating employees throughout the agency. Such a relocation has meant that even experienced staff have been placed in positions for which they lack job training, experience, and possibly suitability for the position. As a result of these personnel dislocations and budget cuts, there were long delays in the release of the detailed reports and public-use data products from the census, with some reports delayed until 1985. In addition, although Public Law 94-52 requires a mid-decade census to be conducted in 1985 (and every 10 years thereafter), funds for this program have not been made available since 1980. In 1985, there was no mid-decade census, and there are no plans as of this writing to conduct one in 1995. This program would have produced small-area data on relatively small subpopulations, including the elderly, on a quinquennial rather than a decennial basis.

Some reports from the 1980 census of interest to researchers in the field of aging were also cancelled. The most important examples are two reports on the older population, one of which would have provided detail on population characteristics of the elderly and the other on their housing characteristics. Other reports that would have produced information on the elderly population along with more general information have been cancelled. These include reports on minority populations, the characteristics of the poverty population, and the sources and structure of household and family income.

Because of a reduction of $1 million in the amount originally proposed for the Survey of Income and Program Participation (SIPP), the sample size of the survey has been reduced by 22.5 percent. A loss of precision of the estimates derived from the survey will result, particularly in the case of small subpopulations such as the elderly.

NATIONAL CENTER FOR HEALTH STATISTICS

In general, the major adjustment made by the National Center for Health Statistics in response to budget reductions has been to stretch out the frequency of its data collections. With respect to the elderly, a major example of this phenomenon is the National Nursing Home Survey, one of four major surveys of health care providers conducted by the Center. Prior to 1980, the frequency of this survey was every three years. Its most recent administration, in 1985, followed a gap of eight years. The next data collection for this survey is currently planned to begin in 1991, but it will be combined with other data collections to be conducted on an ongoing basis. The periodicity of other surveys conducted by the Center has also been decreased, including the National Ambulatory Medical Care Survey, the National Master Facility Inventory, the National Medical Care Utilization and Expenditure Survey, and the National Health and Nutrition Examination Survey. In addition, four medical care provider surveys are slated to be combined into one. Data on the elderly, as well as the rest of the population, will be affected by these changes. The National Ambulatory Medical Care survey serves as the only national source of information on the characteristics of ambulatory medical care received by the elderly (and others) in physicians' offices. The National Master Facility Inventory is the only national source of information on the number of nursing home beds.

The National Health and Nutrition Examination Survey has been stretched out from a planned 5-year cycle to a 10-year one. NHANES is the only national survey that actually includes physical examination of the respondent. The lengthening of the periodicity will create gaps in knowledge of the changing nutritional and health practices of the population.

In 1985 the sample size of the National Health Interview Survey was cut by one-fourth for budgetary reasons; it would have been cut by one-half had NCHS not been able to find reimbursable funding from another agency. To cope with the effects of reduced funding again in the fiscal 1986 budget, and with the 4.7 percent sequestration in the fiscal 1986 budget imposed by the Gramm-Rudman-Hollings Law, NCHS cut the 1986 sample by one-quarter. These cuts will affect the reliability of statistics on subpopulations typically covered in this survey. For 1987, funding was provided for only half the sample, but additional funds from the National Cancer Institute for a supplement on cancer made it possible to conduct a survey on a full sample. In future years, NCHS plans to fund this survey only at the half-sample level, with funding for larger samples to be sought from interested agencies.

NATIONAL CENTER FOR HEALTH SERVICES RESEARCH

While the National Center for Health Services Research does not engage in routine data collection activities similar to those conducted by the other federal agencies discussed in this appendix, it does rely heavily on data sets generated and maintained by such agencies in the conduct of its extramural research program. Such data sets typically constitute the data on which its funded research studies are based. Hence, reductions in sample size, periodicity, and the quality of surveys and administrative records available to the Center affect the nature of the research that can be performed and thus the adequacy of the information available for policy development. In addition, the Center's total budget for any one fiscal year affects the amount of research that can be supported. Since 1973, when the budget was $58 million, it decreased each year until 1982, when it reached $10 million. Since 1985 the budget has risen to the high teens, which is low compared with the early 1970s, and even lower when considered in constant dollars.

Currently, the Center is conducting a new medical expenditure survey, called the National Medical Expenditure Survey, for which it received initial planning funds in fiscal 1986. The design, conduct, and analysis of the NMES is expected to take about five years.

HEALTH CARE FINANCING ADMINISTRATION

The Health Care Financing Administration cosponsored, with the Office of the Assistant Secretary for Planning and Evaluation, the 1982 National Long-Term Care Survey, a unique source of information about the major source of health care costs for the elderly. To reduce initial costs, the size of the survey was reduced to approximately 6,300 noninstitutionalized persons with an impairment. This reduction eliminated coverage of the nonelderly impaired population in long-term care facilities. Although originally designed as a longitudinal survey, in 1982 it was decided to conduct it as a one-time survey because of the high costs of longitudinal surveys. In 1984, however, a decision was made to reinterview the original sample and expand that sample to include (a) people who in 1982 were not functionally impaired, (b) the population that was impaired and institutionalized in 1982, and (c) people who became eligible for Medicare on the basis of age between 1982 and 1984. The 1984 survey was cosponsored by HCFA and the National Center for Health Services Research. As a result of the sequencing of these decisions, the costs associated with following up the sample will actually be greater, and segments of the original sample may be lost.

NATIONAL INSTITUTE OF MENTAL HEALTH

In fiscal 1986, the National Mental Health Statistical Program budget was reduced by 27 percent, followed by an additional reduction in fiscal 1987. The Survey and Reports Branch experienced a decrease of 42 percent in research contract and direct operations funds from fiscal years 1985 to 1987, followed by level funding in fiscal 1988. Affected programs include facility and patient surveys, statistical improvement technical assistance, and applied demographic research. These budget reductions necessitated a change in the periodicity of the facility survey from two to four years, and a change in the periodicity of the patient survey from five to eight years. In addition, the capacity to provide timely data will be diminished, as will the capability to collaborate with the states, local providers, and the mental health community.

SOURCES OF INFORMATION

In addition to conversations with staff in the respective agencies, much of the material in this appendix has been drawn from four reports examining trends in federal statistical programs in recent years:

James R. Storey. *Recent Changes in the Availability of Federal Data on the Aged.* The Gerontological Society of America. Washington, D.C. February 11, 1985.

James R. Storey. *Availability of Federal Data on the Aged: Recent Changes and Future Concerns.* The Gerontological Society of America. Washington, D.C. June 3, 1986.

U.S. Congress, House of Representatives, Committee on Government Operations. *The Federal Statistical System: 1980 to 1985.* 98th Congress, Second Session. November 1984.

U.S. Congress, House of Representatives, Committee on Government Operations. *An Update on the Status of Major Federal Statistical Agencies: Fiscal Year 1986.* 99th Congress, First Session. May 1985.

Appendix C
Descriptions of Data Bases Mentioned in the Panel's Recommendations

The material in this appendix was derived from the Inventory of Data Sets Related to the Health of the Elderly, which was prepared as background for the panel and published in Senate Hearings on Statistical Policy for an Aging America (U.S. Congress, Senate 1986). More detailed information can be found in the inventory. The data base descriptions in the inventory were prepared by agency personnel responsible for the data bases. The data bases and the pages where their descriptions can be found are shown below:

REFERENCE

U.S. Congress, Senate
   1986   *Statistical Policy for an Aging Society.* Joint Hearing of
       the Subcommittee on Energy, Nuclear Proliferation, and
       Government Processes and the Subcommittee on Aging,
       Committee on Governmental Affairs. 99th Congress, 2nd
       Session. Washington, D.C.

TITLE: **Continuous Work History Sample (CWHS)**

SPONSOR: Social Security Administration (SSA), Department of Health and Human Services (DHHS)

YEARS OF DATA COLLECTION: Detailed annual earnings data are currently available for the period 1951-82. Some 1983 data should be available in late 1985. Files are updated annually with a 1- or 2-year lag for accounting and computer processes.

PURPOSE: The CWHS evolved at SSA as the best way of collecting demographic, earnings, employment, and benefit data for use in program research. The files are also used in actuarial activities, the Trustee's Report, and Trust Fund transfers.

DESIGN: The CWHS is a sample data set of administrative records, not a survey. The universe of the data set is all issued social security numbers (SSNs). The CWHS extracts data based on the serial digits of the SSN, usually at a 1% level. The CWHS currently consists of approximately 2.9 million SSNs. The data set is longitudinal in several of its data files. Annual earnings data are available starting in 1951.

CONTENT: The information collected is basically that which SSA needs to administer its retirement program. Data are collected from the:

SS-5	W-2(W-3)	SS-4	1040 Schedule C
Year of birth	Wages	Coded Standard	Self-employed
Race	Type of	Industrial Class	(FICA only)
Sex	employment	State, county	
Place of birth		of employer	

The data are supplemented from various SSA claims forms. Earnings and claims data are collected annually.

TITLE: **County and City Data Book (CCDB)**

SPONSOR: Bureau of Census

YEARS OF DATA COLLECTION: Publication produced roughly every 5 years, though data are collected and processed continuously. CCDB 1983 is the most current edition; next edition is projected for 1987.

PURPOSE: To provide statistical information for states, counties, and cities on subjects such as population, vital statistics, housing, and income.

DESIGN: Data are for geographic units in the United States, compiled from a number of sources.

CONTENT: Continuous collection of county- and city-level data. Information is processed as various data series are produced. Therefore some data are annual, some periodic, and some once in a decade.

PUBLIC-USE DATA TAPES: County and City Data Book 1983 (most recent), CO-STAT 1 (County Statistics 1), County and City Data Book floppy disks.

TITLE: **Decennial Census of Population and Housing**

SPONSOR: Bureau of the Census

YEARS OF DATA COLLECTION: Every 10 years since 1790; the twentieth census was conducted as of April 1, 1980.

PURPOSE: The Constitution mandates that a census be taken every 10 years to provide a basis for reapportioning seats in the House of Representatives.

DESIGN: In the 1980 census, each household in the country received one of two versions of the census questionnaire: a short form containing a limited number of basic population and housing questions or a long form containing these questions as well as a number of additional questions. Two sampling rates were used for the long form. For most of the country, one in every six households (about 17 percent) received the long form or sample questionnaire; in counties, incorporated places and functioning minor civil divisions estimated to have fewer than 2,500 inhabitants, every other household (50 percent) received the sample questionnaire to enhance the reliability of sample data in small areas.

CONTENT: The information collected describes the basic demographic and housing characteristics of the population. There are some comparability problems between censuses because of changes in definitions and procedures. A section on comparability is included in most reports.

PUBLIC-USE DATA TAPES: Available for a sample for 1940, 1950, and 1960. Basic record tapes available for 1970 and 1980 censuses.

TITLE: **Estate/Personal Wealth File**

SPONSOR: Internal Revenue Service (IRS)

YEARS OF DATA COLLECTION: Micro data files have been completed for estate tax returns filed in 1963, 1966, 1970, 1973, 1977, and for 1982 through 1984. Currently, the study is conducted annually. Data on personal wealth were published most recently in the winter 1984-1985 Bulletin; more complete data will be released in winter 1986-1987.

PURPOSE: Collection of data from federal estate tax returns for the purpose of tax administration and for use in the production of personal wealth estimates.

DESIGN: Sample of estate tax returns filed each year. Sample size varies from year to year. Sample based on year of death, age at death, and size of gross estate.

CONTENT: Identifying information, demographic information, asset amounts, liabilities, deductions, net worth, estate tax computation.

Periodically, information on beneficiaries and amounts of bequests are collected.

PUBLIC-USE DATA TAPES: Can be purchased for the years 1973, 1977, 1982, 1983, and 1984.

TITLE: **Linked Medicare Use—NCHS Mortality Statistics File**

SPONSOR: Health Care Financing Administration (HCFA), Department of Health and Human Service (DHHS)

YEARS OF DATA COLLECTION: 1979.

PURPOSE: To study the relation of use of Medicare-covered services to cause of death.

DESIGN: The Medicare utilization and enrollment information in the Continuous Medicare History Sample was linked to the mortality statistics file of the National Center for Health Statistics for a 5% random sample of Medicare enrollees who died in 1979. Of the 70,000 decedents, records were linked for 94%.

CONTENT: Use and cost of Medicare-covered benefits (hospital, physician, home health, skilled nursing facility, hospital outpatient) linked to death certificate data including cause of death. Detail contained in descriptions of Continuous Medicare History File and Mortality Statistics file.

TITLE: **Longitudinal Study of Aging (LSOA)**

SPONSOR: National Center for Health Statistics (NCHS), Department of Health and Human Services (DHHS)

YEARS OF DATA COLLECTION: Baseline survey, 1984. First reinterview, 1986. Record linkage biannually.

PURPOSE: Study changes in functional status. Develop transitional probability models. Study relationship between social and health factors and death.

DESIGN: The Longitudinal Study on Aging is a prospective study based on respondents to the Supplement on Aging, a special set of questions added to the National Health Interview Survey in 1984. Thus the base is a national probability sample of people age 55 and older living in the community. All respondents will be followed by linkage with death records through the National Death Index.

Respondents age 65 and older will be followed by linkage with Medicare records. Respondents age 70 and older will be reinterviewed by telephone.

CONTENT: Interview will focus on changes in functioning, care giving, and living arrangements.

TITLE: **Master Provider of Services File**

SPONSOR: Health Care Financing Administration (HCFA), Department of Health and Human Services (DHHS)

YEARS OF DATA COLLECTION: Reflects the Medicare recertification cycle—from one to three years depending on type of institution. Updated daily on a flow basis.

PURPOSE: To automate the provider certification activity.

DESIGN: All Medicare and Medicaid participating institutional providers.

CONTENT: Provider characteristics:

- Name and address
- Medicare provider number
- Staff size
- Bed size
- Services authorized
- Accreditation
- County, Metropolitan Statistical Area codes

The file is produced from the Medicare/Medicaid Automated Certification System (MMACS).

TITLE: **Medicaid Tape-To-Tape Project**

SPONSOR: Health Care Financing Administration (HCFA), Department of Health and Human Services (DHHS)

YEARS OF DATA COLLECTION: 1980-1982 data from the five participating states have been collected and uniform files completed.

1983-1984 data from participating states are being collected at this time.

PURPOSE: This project was initiated to expand the agency's ability to collect data to analyze the Medicaid program.

DESIGN: The main data base consists of 100% data from five participating states (California, Georgia, Michigan, New York, and Tennessee) in uniform codes and formats. States send their Medicaid Management Information System (MMIS) tapes, which are edited into a comparable format for analysis.

CONTENT: Uniform files are produced for each participating state and year. Separate files are maintained for enrollment, claims, and provider data. Claims, provider, and reimbursements can be linked to the Medicaid enrollee who received the service, and to the provider who furnished it.

TITLE: **Medicare Annual Summary: Person Summary File**

SPONSOR: Health Care Financing Administration (HCFA), Department of Health and Human Services (DHHS)

PURPOSE: The summary file is used to produce statistical reports by age, sex, race, and state of residence, showing number of persons receiving reimbursed Medicare services and amounts reimbursed by type of service.

DESIGN: 5% sample of aged Medicare population based on Social Security number. 25% sample of disabled Medicare population based on Social Security number.

CONTENT: The file is based on bills for the sample population. It shows utilization, charges, and reimbursements by type of service for each person using reimbursed services.

TITLE: Medicare Enrollment File

SPONSOR: Health Care Financing Administration (HCFA), Department of Health and Human Services (DHHS)

YEARS OF DATA COLLECTION: Continuous file beginning with inception of Medicare program, July 1, 1966.

PURPOSE: To maintain information on the demographic and entitlement status of Medicare enrollees, used in the administration of the Medicare program.

DESIGN: All Medicare enrollees.

CONTENT: State and county of residence of Medicare enrollees and type of enrollment (i.e., Part A and/or Part B). Date of birth, sex, race.

TITLE: Medicare History Sample—1974 and Later

SPONSOR: Health Care Financing Administration (HCFA), Department of Health and Human Services (DHHS)

YEARS OF DATA COLLECTION: The file is updated annually. At present the years 1974-1981 are completed.

PURPOSE: The Medicare History Sample was developed to provide a longitudinal person-based data file for statistical research.

DESIGN: The Medicare History File is a 5% sample of all Medicare utilization records based on terminal digits of the Medicare claim number. It is a longitudinal file by person that is updated periodically to include records filed late and to maintain currency by year of medical service.

CONTENT: The file contains demographic data, eligibility data, and Medicare utilization information for a 5% sample of beneficiaries. Records for each stay in hospital or in an extended care facility are added once each year. Summary records for the year are created from physican payment records, home health bills, and outpatient bills and included annually. The utilization data include charge amounts, type of service, dates of service, and diagnoses.

TITLE: **Medicare Part B (SMI) 5-Percent Sample Bill Summary Record**

SPONSOR: Health Care Financing Administration (HCFA), Department of Health and Human Services (DHHS)

YEARS OF DATA COLLECTION: 1976-83—tapes completed, analytic studies ongoing. 1984—ongoing; budgeted and planned.

PURPOSE: To obtain timely data on the amount, type, place, and cost of health care services used under the Supplementary Medical Insurance (SMI Part B) Program.

DESIGN: A 5% sample of SMI bills is selected based on the beneficiary's health insurance claim number. It is linked to the Health Insurance Master File for additional beneficiary and provider information.

CONTENT: Provides information identifying the beneficiary, the physician/supplier, total charges, and reimbursements, as well as data on type and place of service.

TITLE: **Medicare Reimbursement by State and County**

SPONSOR: Health Care Financing Administration (HCFA), Department of Health and Human Services (DHHS)

YEARS OF DATA COLLECTION: Annually since July 1, 1966.

PURPOSE: To measure utilization of Medicare services.

DESIGN: All bills reimbursed under the Medicare program are allocated to residence of the beneficiary annually.

CONTENT: The file shows reimbursement for residents of each state and county enrolled in the Medicare program, as a grand total and separately for the Hospital Insurance Program (HI) and the Supplementary Medical Insurance Program (SMI).

TITLE: National Ambulatory Medical Care Survey
           (NAMCS)

SPONSOR: National Center for Health Statistics (NCHS), Department of Health and Human Services (DHHS)

YEARS OF DATA COLLECTION: Data collected annually from 1973 through 1981. Repeated in 1985 and scheduled on a triennial basis thereafter. 1985 data will be released in fall 1986.

PURPOSE: To provide general purpose statistics describing the public's use of office-based physician services, the health problems presented to physicians by ambulatory patients, and the diagnostic and therapeutic services received.

DESIGN: Universe: all patient visits to office-based physicians in contiguous United States. Multistage sample design including 3,000 to 5,000 physicians in about 80 geographic areas. Probability sample, response of approximately 75%. Sample size 3,000 physicians, 50,000 patient visits through 1981. Sample size in 1985: 5,000 physicians, 75,000 visits.

CONTENT: Information includes patient age, sex, race, ethnicity, and reason for visit; physician's diagnostic and therapeutic services ordered or provided; diagnosis and disposition decision and drugs prescribed. Variations from year to year are slight.

PUBLIC-USE DATA TAPES: For all years in which survey has been completed.

TITLE: National Data Base on Aging

SPONSOR: Administration on Aging (AoA), Department of Health and Human Services (DHHS)

YEARS OF DATA COLLECTION: Annually since 1981.

PURPOSE: The National Data Base on Aging is a voluntary annual survey that collects information at the national level about the network of state and area agency on aging programs.

DESIGN: Initial questionnaires were mailed to all 57 state units and 666 area agencies in September 1981. State units are surveyed annually. Updates for area agencies are made from a systematic 1/3 sample in each subsequent year, with a 65% response rate in 1984.

CONTENT: The data collection included questions on the staffing of the agencies, the types of funding used, and the characteristics of service providers, services provided, and service recipients.

PUBLIC-USE DATA TAPES: Accessed through the National Data Base on Aging.

TITLE: **National Death Index (NDI)**

SPONSOR: National Center for Health Statistics (NCHS), Department of Health and Human Services (DHHS)

YEARS OF DATA COLLECTION: The NDI file contains 10.3 million death records for 1979-1983. Deaths are added to the file annually, approximately 12-14 months after the end of a calendar year. About 2 million records are added each year.

PURPOSE: The National Death Index (NDI) is a computerized central file of death record information. It is compiled from magnetic tapes submitted to the National Center for Health Statistics (NCHS) by the state vital statistics offices. These tapes contain a standard set of identifying information for each decedent, beginning with deaths occurring in 1979.

Investigators conducting prospective and retrospective studies can use the NDI to determine whether persons in their studies may have died, and if so, be provided with the names of the states in which those deaths occurred, the dates of death, and the corresponding death certificate numbers. The NDI user can then arrange with the appropriate state offices to obtain copies of death certificates or specific statistical information such as cause of death.

DESIGN: The NDI file contains identifying death record information for virtually all deaths in the United States, Puerto Rico, and the Virgin Islands.

CONTENT: The identifying information on the NDI file is provided to NCHS on magnetic tapes submitted by the state vital statistics offices via contractual agreements. The items of information are: state of death, death certificate number, date of death, first and last name, middle initial, father's surname, social security number, date of birth, race, sex, marital status, state of residence, state of birth, age at death.

TITLE: **National Health Interview Survey (NHIS): Core Questionnaire**

SPONSOR: National Center for Health Statistics (NCHS), Department of Health and Human Services (DHHS)

YEARS OF DATA COLLECTION: Annually since 1957.

PURPOSE: To provide data on the incidence of acute conditions, limitation of activity, persons injured, hospitalizations, disability days, dental visits, physician visits, and the prevalence of selected chronic conditions.

DESIGN: The NHIS is a continuing, nationwide, household interview survey. A probability sample of households in the civilian noninstitutionalized population of the United States is interviewed each week by interviewers from the Bureau of the Census. The sample consists of about 50,000 households representing about 130,000 persons. The NHIS "core" is not longitudinal and historically has not been linked to other files. An NHIS/National Death Index linkage capability was made possible after the 1984 NHIS survey year. In the future, beginning at the conclusion of the 1987 NHIS survey year, linkage capabilities will also exist between the NHIS, the National Medical Care Expenditure Survey, and the National Family Growth Survey.

CONTENT: The NHIS provides current information on the amount, distribution, and effects of illness and disability in the United States, and the services rendered for or because of such conditions. The NHIS "core" has been virtually unchanged from year to year.

PUBLIC-USE DATA TAPES: Available through 1982.

TITLE: **National Health Interview Survey (NHIS): Supplements**

SPONSOR: National Center for Health Statistics (NCHS), Department of Health and Human Services (DHHS)

YEARS OF DATA COLLECTION: See Content.

PURPOSE: To provide data, in addition to the basic NHIS data, on special topic areas pertinent to the aging population, such as living arrangements, activities of daily living (ADL), instrumental activities of daily living (IADL), retirement status, support systems, etc.

DESIGN: The universe studied are those persons in the U.S. non-institutionalized civilian population in the age categories of interest, as represented by persons in those age categories in the NHIS probability sample of households.

CONTENT: Supplements to the NHIS have been conducted annually for the past 20 years. Topics of coverage in the supplement vary from year to year and may or may not apply to the aging population. Among those that include or are designed specifically for an aging population are:

> Arthritis—1969, 1976.
> Residential mobility—1979, 1980.
> Hearing aid—1971, 1977, 1979.
> Visual and hearing impairment—1971, 1977, 1984.
> Edentulousness—1971.
> Home care—1979, 1980.
> Supplement on aging—1984.

TITLE: **National Health Interview Survey (NHIS): Supplement on Aging (SOA), 1984**

SPONSOR: National Center for Health Statistics (NCHS), Department of Health and Human Services (DHHS)

YEARS OF DATA COLLECTION: 1984.

PURPOSE: The National Health Interview Survey (NHIS) is a

multipurpose national survey that is the principal source of information on the health of the civilian, noninstitutionalized population of the United States. It provides current statistical information on the amount, distribution, and effects of illness and disabilities in the United States and the services rendered for or because of such conditions. The Supplement on Aging (SOA) provides data on functional limitations and the health and social care received by the elderly, noninstitutionalized population, to complement the National Nursing Home Survey.

DESIGN: Persons ages 55 years and older in the 1984 NHIS household sample, which has a response rate of 97%, were selected for the SOA sample: 50% of NHIS respondents ages 55-64 and 100% of persons ages 65 and older were included. Response rate to the SOA was also 97%.

CONTENT: Health status, functional ability, health and community service utilization, employment status, social activities, family relationships and social support, housing characteristics and living arrangements, and existence of health conditions specific to the elderly population. The information in the supplement for each person can be associated with the basic health and condition information in the NHIS core questionnaire.

PUBLIC-USE DATA TAPES: Expected to be available in 1986.

TITLE: **National Health and Nutrition Examination Survey (NHANES I)**

SPONSOR: National Center for Health Statistics (NCHS), Department of Health and Human Services (DHHS)

YEARS OF DATA COLLECTION: 1971 to 1975. NHANES II was conducted from 1976 to 1980. NHANES III planned to start 1988.

PURPOSE: Established under the National Health Survey Act of 1956 to obtain those kinds of health data optimally obtained by direct physical examinations and physiological and biochemical measurements. Measures and monitors health and nutritional status of the U.S. population. Permits estimation of the prevalence of certain diseases and the distributions of a broad variety of health-related measurements.

DESIGN: Probability sample of the U.S. civilian noninstitutionalized population ages 1 through 74 years. Cross-sectional study of 31,973 persons of whom 23,808 were examined. Composed of two overlapping sets of examination components referred to as the nutrition examination and the detailed medical examination. Six distinct probability samples were contained within the overall survey. This study was used as the baseline for a later study called the NHANES I Epidemiologic Follow-up Survey.

CONTENT: Demographic information; medical histories; dietary information; electrocardiograms; body measurements; dermatological and ophthalmological examinations; general medical examination; hematological, blood chemistry, and urological laboratory determinations. In the detailed medical examination, additional data were collected on a subsample of adults 25-74 years by supplementary questionnaires concerning arthritis, respiratory conditions, and cardiovascular conditions; an extended medical examination, x-rays of the chest for heart size and pathology as well as lung volume and pathology; x-rays of the hip, sacroiliac, and knee joints for assessment of arthritic and related changes; spirometry and additional laboratory determinations.

PUBLIC-USE DATA TAPES: Data tapes are available on virtually all the information collected in NHANES I. Data collected in the HANES surveys can be located by means of HINDEX, available in hard copy or on a floppy diskette. HINDEX has been released in three volumes: one indexes the data items in alphabetical sort by data category; the second is an alphabetical sort by data field; and the third, a numerical sort by tape and position field.

TITLE: **NHANES I Epidemiologic Follow-up Study: Initial Follow-up, 1982-84**

SPONSORS: National Center for Health Statistics (NCHS) with National Institute on Aging and other Institutes

YEARS OF DATA COLLECTIONS: The NHANES I Epidemiologic Follow-up Study: initial follow-up 1982-84; continued follow-up of the elderly 1985-86; continued follow-up of total sample 1986-87; data tapes will be available in 1990.

PURPOSE: Identify chronic disease risk factors associated with morbidity and mortality; ascertain changes in risk factors, morbidity, functional limitation and institutionalization between NHANES I and the follow-up recontacts; and map the natural history of chronic diseases and functional impairments in an aging population.

DESIGN: The baseline survey, the first National Health and Nutrition Examination Survey (NHANES) conducted by NCHS from 1971 to 1975 was a probability sample of the civilian noninstitutionalized coterminous U.S. population ages 1-74 years. The population of the follow-up study includes the 14,407 persons who were ages 25-74 at the time they were examined in the original NHANES I Survey.

CONTENT: Demographic characteristics, labor force participation, income, acute and chronic conditions, activity limitations, impairments, cognitive impairment, usual activity, changes in morbidity and self-perceived health, activities of daily living, inpatient health care utilization (hospital, nursing home, etc.).

PUBLIC-USE DATA TAPES: Initial follow-up: tapes available in 1987. Continue follow-up of elderly: tapes available in 1989. Continued follow-up of total sample: tapes available in 1990.

TITLE: **National Master Facility Inventory (NMFI)**

SPONSOR: National Center for Health Statistics (NCHS), Department of Health and Human Services (DHHS)

YEARS OF DATA COLLECTION: Data were collected for the following years: 1963, 1967,1969, 1971, 1973, 1976, 1978, 1980, 1982. The first report on data from the 1982 survey was published in September 1985; the second will be published during 1986. Because an evaluation of the NMFI program is under way, the inventory will not be conducted before 1988.

PURPOSE: The NMFI has two basic purposes. It is an important national source of statistics on the number, type, and geographic distribution of inpatient facilities in the United States. In addition, it serves as the universe from which probability samples are selected for conducting sample surveys.

DESIGN: The NMFI is a comprehensive file of all facilities in the United States with three or more beds that provide medical, nursing, personal, or custodial care to groups of unrelated persons on an inpatient basis. Facilities are categorized into three broad types: hospitals, nursing and related care homes, and other custodial or remedial care facilities.

CONTENT: Basically, the types of data collected for the three categories of facilities are: ownership; major type of service; number of beds; patient census; number of admissions, discharges, and deaths; and information about staffing, revenue, and expenses.

PUBLIC-USE DATA TAPES: For all years.

TITLE:	**National Medical Care Expenditures Survey (NMCES), 1977-78, and National Medical Expenditure Survey (NMES, planned for 1987)**
SPONSORS:	National Center for Health Services Research and Health Care Technology Assessment (NCHSR) and National Center for Health Statistics (NCHS) (NMCES only), Health Care Financing Administration (HCFA) (NMES only), Department of Health and Human Services (DHHS)

YEARS OF DATA COLLECTION: NMCES consists of six rounds of data collection covering an 18-month period between 1977 and part of 1978. A 1987 National Medical Expenditure Survey (NMES) is planned jointly with NCHSR and the Health Care Financing Administration. The household sample is expected to have about 14,000 households including oversamples of blacks, Hispanics, low-income people and people with functional limitations. The Institutional Population Component sample will include about 13,000 clients of nursing and personal care homes, psychiatric hospitals, and facilities for the mentally retarded.

PURPOSE: The National Medical Care Expenditures Survey was designed to provide a comprehensive statistical picture of how health services are used and paid for in the United States.

DESIGN: NMCES is a one-time panel sample that interviewed about 40,000 persons in 14,000 randomly selected households in the civilian, noninstitutionalized population. The sample design is a stratified, multistage, area probability sample that allows for the determination of approximately unbiased estimates of health parameters at the national level. Respondents were interviewed six times over an 18-month period during 1977 and 1978. The survey was complemented by additional surveys of physicians and health care facilities providing care to household members during 1977 and of employers and insurance companies responsible for their insurance coverage. The principal NMCES response rate was 82%, defined as the proportion of eligible first-round reporting units that responded to all rounds of interviewing.

CONTENT: Data collected includes but is not limited to: expenditures and sources of payment for all major forms of medical care; sociodemographic and economic characteristics of respondents; insurance coverage of respondents; information from medical providers about respondents; and access to medical care.

PUBLIC-USE DATA TAPES: NMCES available for person-based information and on events of medical care. Additional public-use files on insurance coverage, employer characteristics, and episodes of illness will be available in the future.

TITLE: **National Medical Care Utilization and Expenditure Survey (NMCUES), 1980**

SPONSORS: National Center for Health Statistics (NCHS) and Health Care Financing Administration (HCFA)

YEARS OF DATA COLLECTION: 1980.

PURPOSE: NMCUES is designed to be directly responsive to the continuing need for statistical information on the health care expenditures associated with health services utilization for the entire U.S. population. Cycle 1 was designed and conducted in collaboration with the Health Care Financing Administration to provide detailed utilization and expenditure data for persons in the Medicare and Medicaid populations. NMCUES will produce estimates over time for evaluation of the impact of legislation and programs on health status, costs, utilization and illness-related behavior in the medical care delivery system.

Cycle 1 was composed of several related surveys. The household portion of the survey consisted of a national survey of the civilian noninstitutionalized population and a separate survey of the Medicaid-eligible populations of the states of New York, California, Texas, and Michigan. These two surveys each consisted of five interviews over a period of about 15 months to obtain information on medical care utilization, expenditures, and other health-related information. A third survey, an administrative records survey, was designed to verify the eligibility status of the household survey respondents for the Medicare and Medicaid programs. It also checked insurance claims filed with the national Medicare program and Medicaid programs in each of the four states for persons in the sample of Medicaid eligibles.

DESIGN: The national Cycle 1 household survey comprised persons residing in about 6,000 households. The sample for this survey was a multistage area probability sample drawn from 106 primary sampling units representing the 50 states and the District of Columbia. The state Medicaid household survey sample consisted of about 1,000 families in each of the four states; these families were selected with a known probability of selection from the state Medicaid enrollment lists. Thus, the total sample for the survey was about 10,000 households.

An overall response rate of 89.4% was achieved in the first interview for both household surveys in Cycle 1: for the national survey the response rate was 91.4%, and for the state Medicaid survey the rate was 86.7%. Attrition over the course of interviewing resulted in final response rates of 84.9% for the national household survey and 76.1% for the state Medicaid household survey.

CONTENT: Questionnaires for the household surveys were designed to obtain some information on a repeated basis throughout the survey and some information only one time. The repetitive core of questions for Cycle 1 included health insurance coverage, episodes of illness, the number of bed days, restricted activity days, hospital admissions, physician and dental visits, other medical care encounters, and purchases of prescribed medicines. For each contact with the medical care system, data were obtained on the nature of the health conditions, characteristics of the provider, services provided, charges, sources, and amounts of payment. Questions asked only once included data on access to medical care services, limitation of activities, occupation, income, and other sociodemographic characteristics.

PUBLIC-USE DATA TAPES: Available.

TITLE: National Mortality Statistics File

SPONSOR: National Center for Health Statistics (NCHS), Department of Health and Human Services (DHHS)

YEARS OF DATA COLLECTION: Data are collected annually. Data through 1983 are available and will be published in annual volumes of *Vital Statistics of the United States, Vol. II*, "Mortality," Parts A and B. Summary counts of deaths by age, race, sex, and cause are available on a current basis in *Monthly Vital Statistics Report*, as are provisional monthly counts of deaths by cause.

PURPOSE:To produce uniform national, state, and local data on numbers of deaths, causes of death, and sociodemographic characteristics of decedents.

DESIGN: Mortality data include all deaths (approximately 2 million) occurring annually within the United States reported to state vital registration offices.   In 1972, a 50% sample of mortality data was used; generally, however, 100% of deaths are included. Data are collected annually. Data are available for the entire U.S. annually since 1933 and for selected states since 1900.

CONTENT: Demographic and medical information is coded from information reported on the death certificate including residence, age, race, sex, underlying cause of death, and multiple causes of death.

PUBLIC-USE DATA TAPES: Available for data years 1963-83.

TITLE: National Nursing Home Survey (NNHS)

SPONSOR: National Center for Health Statistics (NCHS), Department of Health and Human Services (DHHS)

YEARS OF DATA COLLECTION: 1973-74, 1977, 1985, and proposed for 1990.

PURPOSE: To collect data on nursing homes, their services, staffs, and financial characteristics, and on personal and health characteristics of residents and discharges.

DESIGN: Data are collected from a sample of all nursing homes in the coterminous United States (1,200 nursing homes listed in the Master Facility Inventory). Samples in each nursing home are selected of current residents, persons discharged (deceased or alive in the last year), and staff members. Data on residents and discharges are collected by interviewing the nurse who obtains the needed information from the medical records and the next of kin. Estimates are produced for the United States, census regions, and DHHS regions, and in 1977 for five states with the largest nursing home populations.

CONTENT: The survey collects data on characteristics of the facility and its finances, of residents, of discharges, and of staff, as follows:

> *Facility*: size, ownership, Medicare and Medicaid certification, staffing patterns, and services offered.
> *Financial characteristics*: Total expenses and major components of operation.
> *Residents*: Demographic characteristics, living arrangements prior to admission, diagnosis and conditions, functional status, receipt of services (medical, nursing, and therapeutic), cost of care, source of payment.
> *Discharges*: A subset of items collected for current residents available from the record.
> *Staff*: Data varied with survey. In 1985 survey, characteristics of registered nurses—work schedule, experience, activities in facility, demographic characteristics, and salary were collected.
> *Next of kin*: Information about residents' and discharges' living arrangements, health and functional status prior to nursing home admission, lifetime use of nursing home care, Medicaid spend-down.

PUBLIC-USE DATA TAPES: With the exception of individual or establishment identifiers, all data collected are available on the public use data tape.

TITLE: **Statistics of Income: Individual Income Tax Returns**

SPONSOR: Internal Revenue Service (IRS)

YEARS OF DATA COLLECTION: Data are collected for each tax year. Individual income tax data are currently available for tax years 1913 through 1983. These data will continue to be collected, processed, and published in future years.

PURPOSE: The production of individual income tax statistics was authorized by the Revenue Act of 1916. Statistics of income data are used by a variety of agencies for tax system and economic analyses.

DESIGN: Statistics of income data are estimated from a stratified probability sample of income tax returns and supporting schedules filed with the Internal Revenue Service. The sample is based on such criteria as: principal business activity; presence or absence of a schedule; state from which filed; size of adjusted gross income (or deficit) or largest of specific income (or loss) items; total assets or size of business and farm receipts. The sample size alternates from 80,000 to 120,000 returns each year, selected from a population of approximately 96 million returns. Special searches are conducted for returns selected so that any bias from nonresponse is minimal. A large proportion of the sample is longitudinal and research on the longitudinal design of the sample is being conducted. The individual income tax returns sample does not make use of data linked to other files, however, certain other statistics of income studies do use linked data files.

CONTENT: Data relative to taxpayers' income, exemptions, deductions, credits, and tax are collected. Due to changes in tax laws, items collected vary from tax year to tax year.

PUBLIC-USE DATA TAPES: Available on a reimbursable basis.

TITLE: **Survey of Income and Program Participation (SIPP)**

SPONSOR: Bureau of the Census

YEARS OF DATA COLLECTION: The initial interviews for the 1984 panel began in October 1983. Seven of nine proposed waves of the 1984 panel have been completed. In February 1985 a new panel began and three waves of interviewing have been completed. A new panel will be implemented each February. The first five quarterly reports—third quarter 1983, fourth quarter 1983, first quarter 1984, second quarter 1984, and third quarter 1985—have been released.

PURPOSE: The objectives of SIPP include the collection of data on cash and noncash income for the purpose of studying the efficiency of transfer and service programs, the estimation of future program costs and coverage, and the assessment of the effects of proposed policy changes. SIPP will also satisfy the need for improved data on the economic situation of persons and families in the United States to produce improved estimates of the distribution of income, poverty, and wealth.

DESIGN: SIPP started in October 1983 as an ongoing nationally representative survey of the Bureau of the Census with one sample panel of approximately 21,000 households in 174 primary sample units selected to represent the noninstitutional population of the United States. The sample design is self-weighting.

Each household is interviewed once every 4 months for 2 2/3 years to produce sufficient data for longitudinal analyses while providing a relatively short recall period for reporting monthly income and labor force activity. The reference period for the principal survey items is the four months preceding the interview.

Each February a new panel goes into the field with a sample size of about 15,000 households. Members of each panel go through eight interviews or waves. In order to spread the workload for the field staff, members of each panel are divided into four groups of equal size called rotation groups. Each month in turn one rotation group receives its interview. Thus the four month relevance period is different for each rotation group.

At this time, cross-sectional unit noninterview rates are available for the first two waves of SIPP. Unit noninterview rates provide a measure of the success/failure of the SIPP field work. While refusals are the largest part of the type A rate, it also includes "no one home" and "temporarily absent" households. In Wave 1 (all rotation groups), the mean type A rate was 4.8%; in Wave 2, 3.7%, in Wave 3, 5.6%. The cumulative Type A rate after 3 interviews is approximately 12%.

A study has been implemented to validate electronically reported social security numbers (SSN), to manually search for SSNs not reported correctly, and to use the panel aspect of the SIPP to correct and verify a respondent's SSN. Having established the link for matching activities, work is now proceeding on identifying content and availability of administrative record systems for use in: (a) data augmentation for research and estimates and (b) survey data evaluation.

Another aspect of this work is the development of a demonstration and feasibility study to evaluate SIPP data from Waves 1 and 2 using several federal administrative record systems such as the Master Beneficiary Record (SSA), and the Supplemental Security Record (SSA).

CONTENT: The content of SIPP was developed around a "core" of labor force and income questions designed to measure the economic situation of persons ages 15 and over in the United States. These questions expand the data currently available on the distribution of cash and noncash income and are repeated at *each* interviewing wave.

Specific questions are asked about the types of income received, including transfer payments and noncash benefits from various programs, disability, assets and liabilities, pension coverage, taxes, and many other items, for each month of the reference period, as well as labor force status, which is collected on a weekly basis. A few questions on private health insurance coverage are also included in the core.

The SIPP has been designed to provide a broader context for analysis by adding questions on a variety of topics not covered in the core section. These questions are labeled "fixed topical modules" and are assigned to particular interviewing waves of the survey. For example, questions are asked about health and disability in the third interview of the 1984 panel, and questions are asked about the value of assets and liabilities in the fourth interview of the 1984 panel. If more than one observation is needed, questions on one wave may be repeated on a later wave.

In response to program planning and policy analysis data requirements, the final component of the SIPP content consists of modules of questions designed in consultation with other federal agencies. These variable topical modules are designed to be flexible and to meet immediate policy analysis needs. For example, Wave 4 includes data on pension plan coverage and retirement plans and expectations.

PUBLIC-USE DATA TAPES: SIPP micro data files for Waves 1-4 of the 1984 panel have been released.

TITLE: **Yearly Continuous Disability History Sample (CDHS)**

SPONSOR: Social Security Administration (SSA), Department of Health and Human Services (DHHS)

YEARS OF DATA COLLECTION: Annually since 1975. The latest available file is for 1983.

PURPOSE: To furnish statistics on the operations of the social security disability program and the characteristics of the claimant population.

DESIGN: The CDHS is a yearly 20% simple random sample of initial disability claims processed by the Social Security Administration. The 1983 sample contained approximately 300,000 records. The sample is linked to the Master Beneficiary Record (MBR) and the Summary Earnings Record (SER).

CONTENT: The basic data set comprises: personal characteristics—sex, race, date of birth, occupation; agency decision—allowance/ denial, legal basis, medical diagnosis, onset date; payment history— worker and family payments; annual earnings.

See Division of Disability Studies, Users' Manual for the 1976 Continuous Disability History Sample (CDHS) Restricted Use Data File.

Appendix D
Long-term Health Care Minimum Data Set

The Technical Consultant Panel on the Long-Term Health Care Data Set, National Committee on Vital and Health Statistics, recommends that all public and voluntary reporting systems for long-term health care clients and services collect the following minimum set of information, as specified in the *Long-Term Health Care Minimum Data Set*, National Committee on Vital and Health Statistics, U.S. Department of Health and Human Services, August 1980. DHHS Publication No. (PHS) 80-1158 (p.1).

Demographic Items

1. Personal Identification
2. Sex
3. Birth date
4. Race and ethnicity
   a. Race
   b. Ethnicity
5. Marital status
6. Usual living arrangements
   a. Type
   b. Location
7. Court-ordered constraints
   a. Court-ordered care
   b. Court-ordered guardian

Health Status Items

8. Vision
9. Hearing
10. Communication
    a. Expressive communication
    b. Receptive communication
11. Basic activities of daily living
    a. Bathing and showering
    b. Dressing
    c. Using toilet
    d. Transferring in and out of bed or chair
    e. Continence
    f. Eating
    g. Walking
12. Mobility
13. Adaptive tasks
14. Behavior problems
15. Orientation or memory impairment
16. Disturbance of mood
17. Primary and other significant diagnoses

Service Items

18. Provider identification
    a. Unique number
    b. Location
    c. Type of provider (includes general hospital, specialty hospital, nursing home, residential care facility, hospice, and community-based services)
19. Last principal provider
20. Date of admission or commencement of service
21. Direct services (includes personal care, nursing services, medical services by medical doctor or doctor of osteopathy, other medical services, mental health services, social services, physical therapy, occupational therapy, speech and hearing therapy, vocational rehabilitation, special education, nutritionist services, sheltered employment, homemaker-household services, and transportation)
22. Direct services
23. Charges

24. Discharge or termination of service
     a.   Date
     b.   Status or destination

Procedural Items

25. Date of report
26. Type of report

Appendix E
Acronyms

ADL	Activities of daily living
AFDC	Aid to Families With Dependent Children
AHCA	American Health Care Association
AMA	American Medical Association
ANA	American Nurses Association
ADA	American Dental Association
AOA	Administration on Aging (DHHS)
ASTHO	Association of State and Territorial Health Officers
BLS	Bureau of Labor Statistics
CARE	Comprehensive Assessment and Referral Evaluation
CCDB	City and County Data Book
CDHS	Continuous Disability History Sample
CES-D	Center for Epidemiological Studies - Depression
CON	Certificate of Need
CO-STAT1	County Statistics 1
CPS	Current Population Survey (Census Bureau)
CWHS	Continuous Work History Sample
DECO	Demographic-Economic Model of the Elderly
DHHS	Department of Health and Human Services
DIS	Diagnostic Interview Schedule
DSMIII	Diagnostic and Statistical Manual, 3d ed.
DRG	Diagnosis-related group
DRI	Data Resources, Inc.
ECA	Epidemiologic Catchment Area (NIMH)

EPESE	Established Populations for Epidemiologic Studies of the Elderly (NIA)
FICA	Federal Insured Contributions Act
GHAA	Group Health Association of America
GNP	Gross National Product
HCFA	Health Care Financing Administration (DHHS)
HHA	Home Health Agency
HI	Hospital Insurance Program (Medicare Program, HCFA)
HIAA	Health Insurance Association of America
HINDEX	Index to data collected in the NHANES surveys (NCHS)
HMO	Health Maintenance Organization
IADL	Instrumental activities of daily living
ICD-9-CM	International Classification of Diseases, 9th Revision, Clinical Modification
ICIDH	International Classification of Impairments, Disabilities and Handicaps
IOM	Institute of Medicine (National Academy of Sciences)
IPC	Institutional Population Component (NMES)
IQC	Integrated Quality Control
IRA	Individual retirement account
IRS	Internal Revenue Service
ISHIS	Integrated System of Health Interview Surveys
LTC	Long-term care
LPN	Licensed practical nurse
LRHS	Longitudinal Retirement History Study (SSA)
LSOA	Longitudinal Study of Aging (NCHS)
MADRS	Medicare Automated Data Retrieval System (HCFA)
MAI	Multilevel Assessment Instrument
MEDPAR	Medicare Provider Analysis and Review (HCFA)
MMACS	Medicare/Medicaid Automated Certification System (HCFA)
MMIS	Medicaid Management Information System
MQCS	Medicaid Quality Control System (HCFA)
MSS	Medicare Statistical System (HCFA)
MDM	Macroeconomic-Demographic Model
NACDA	National Archive of Computerized Data on Aging (University of Michigan)
NAMCS	National Ambulatory Medical Care Survey (NCHS)
NASUA	National Association of State Units on Aging
NATCS	National Long-term Care Survey
NCHS	National Center for Health Statistics

NCHSR	National Center for Health Services Research and Health Care Technology Assessment
NDI	National Death Index
NHANES	National Health and Nutrition Examination Survey (NCHS)
NHDS	National Hospital Discharge Survey (NCHS)
NHIS	National Health Interview Survey (NCHS)
NIA	National Institute on Aging ((DHHS)
NIMH	National Institute of Mental Health (DHHS)
NMCES	National Medical Care Expenditures Survey (NCHSR with NCHS)
NMCUES	National Medical Care Utilization and Expenditures Survey (NCHS with HCFA)
NMES	National Medical Expenditure Survey (NCHSR)
NMFI	National Master Facility Inventory (NCHS)
NNHS	National Nursing Home Survey (NCHS)
OARS	Older American Resources and Services (Duke University)
OIRA	Office of Information and Regulatory Affairs (OMB)
OMB	Office of Management and Budget
PHS	Public Health Service (DHHS)
PPO	Preferred provider organization
PPS	Prospective payment system
PRISM	Project to Redesign Information System Management (HCFA)
RAND HIS	RAND Corporation's Health Insurance Study
SHMO	Social Health Maintenance Organization
SIPP	Survey of Income and Program Participation (Bureau of Census)
SMI	Supplementary Medical Insurance (Medicare Program, HCFA)
SNF	Skilled nursing facility
SOA	Supplement on Aging (NHIS, NCHS)
SSA	Social Security Administration
SSN	Social Security number
TEFRA	Tax Equity and Fiscal Responsibility Act
UHDDS	Uniform Hospital Discharge Data Set
VA	Veterans Administration
WHO	World Health Organization

Appendix F
Biographical Sketches

SAM SHAPIRO (Chair) is professor emeritus of health policy and management and past director of the Health Services Research and Development Center in the School of Hygiene and Public Health at Johns Hopkins University. He is a senior member of the Institute of Medicine, a member of the American Epidemiologic Society, and a fellow of the American Public Health Association, the American Statistical Association, the American Association for the Advancement of Science, and the American Heart Association. His fields of interest are biostatistics and epidemiology, and his publications cover such topics as information systems, the organization, distribution, utilization, and quality of care, secondary prevention of breast cancer, coronary heart disease prognosis, and the need for mental health services. He received a B.S. degree from Brooklyn College in 1933 and has carried out graduate study in statistics at Columbia and George Washington Universities.

DAN GERMAN BLAZER II is professor of psychiatry at Duke University Medical Center and adjunct professor of epidemiology at the University of North Carolina. He directs the Affective Disorders Program and the Center for the Study of Depression in the Elderly. He also serves currently as principal investigator of the National Institute on Aging's Established Populations for Epidemiologic Studies in the Elderly project and was previously the principal investigator for the Duke Epidemiological Catchment Area Project. His present work examines the epidemiology of physical and mental health in both clinical and community populations. He received an M.D. degree from the University of Tennessee and also has M.P.H. and Ph.D. degrees in epidemiology from the University of North Carolina.

LAURENCE G. BRANCH is professor of community medicine and public health at Boston University and chairman of the health services section in the School of Public Health. During the deliberations of the panel he was an associate professor at Harvard University and a health policy gerontologist at the Harvard Division on Aging. He received a B.A. in psychology from Marquette University and M.A. and Ph.D. degrees in social psychology from Loyola University. He has been the chairman of the Gerontological Health Section of the American Public Health Association and a member of the 1981 White House Conference on Aging. He has been the director of the Massachusetts Health Care Panel Study, a longitudinal study of community older people, since 1974. His publications clarify the development of disabilities and the use of health and social services by older citizens.

NEAL E. CUTLER is professor of political science and gerontology at the University of Southern California and codirector of the Institute for Advanced Study in Gerontology and Geriatrics at the University's Andrus Gerontology Center. In 1972-1973 he was a Fulbright research fellow at Helsinki University, and in 1979-1980 served as a staff member of the U.S. Senate Special Committee on Aging. He is a fellow of the Gerontological Society of America and a member of the editorial board of the American Society on Aging. He is currently directing the country's first national survey of public knowledge about and perceptions of Alzheimer's disease. He received a Ph.D. in political science from Northwestern University.

DOROTHY M. GILFORD served as study director of the panel's work. Formerly, she served as director of the National Center for Education Statistics and as director of the mathematical sciences division of the Office of Naval Research. Her interests are in research program administration, organization of statistical systems, education administration, education statistics, and human resource statistics. A fellow of the American Statistical Association, she has served as vice president of the association and chairman of its committee on fellows. She is a member of the International Statistics Institute. She received B.S. and M.S. degrees in mathematics from the University of Washington.

JEANNE E. GRIFFITH is a specialist in social legislation at the Congressional Research Service of the Library of Congress. She has served as a survey statistician at the Office of Management and Budget, the Department of Health, Education, and Welfare, and the Bureau of the Census and as a demographer at the Bureau of the Census and for the government of the county of Fairfax, Virginia. Her principal interests have been the relationships between demographic trends and public policy as well as federal statistical policy. She received a B.A. from the College of William and Mary, an M.A. in sociology from the University of Pennsylvania, an M.S. in statistics from George Washington University, and a Ph.D. in sociology from Johns Hopkins University.

ROBERT L. KAHN is a research scientist at the Institute for Social Research of the University of Michigan as well as professor of psychology and of public health at that university. He is a fellow of the American Psychological Association, the American Statistical Association, and the Academy of Behavioral Medicine Research. His research interests began with organizational theory and now emphasize psychosocial factors that influence productive behavior throughout the life course. He received a Ph.D. degree in social psychology from the University of Michigan.

GARY G. KOCH is professor of biostatistics at the School of Public Health, University of North Carolina, where he has served on the faculty since 1968. He received a B.S. in mathematics and an M.S. in industrial engineering from Ohio State University and a Ph.D in statistics from the University of North Carolina. His principal research interest has been the development of statistical methodology for the analysis of categorical data and corresponding applications to a broad range of research settings in the health and social sciences. He served as the editor of *The American Statistician* during 1981-1984. He currently is chairman of the Committee for the American Statistical Association Sesquicentennial in 1989.

JUDITH R. LAVE is professor of health economics at the Graduate School of Public Health, University of Pittsburgh. She received undergraduate training at Queen's University in Canada and a Ph.D. in economics from Harvard University. She has been a faculty member of Carnegie-Mellon University; director of Economic Quantitative Analysis, Office of the Deputy Assistant Secretary for Planning and Evaluation, Department of Health and Human Services; and director of the Office of Research, Health Care Financing Administration.

She has served as a consultant to both private and public agencies and has served on a number of national committees. She is currently a member of the Institute of Medicine's Committee on Health Care for the Homeless and on the Technical Advisory Panel on the Evaluation of the Medicare Prospective Payment System of the Health Care Financing Administration. She is president-elect of the Association for Health Services Research.

DOROTHY P. RICE is professor in residence in the Department of Social and Behavioral Sciences, with joint appointments with the Institute for Health and Aging and the Institute for Health Policy Studies, at the University of California, San Francisco. From 1977 to 1982 she served as director of the National Center for Health Statistics. Previously she served as deputy assistant commissioner for research and statistics of the Social Security Administration. She is a member of the Institute of Medicine, a fellow of the American Statistical Association and the American Public Health Association, and a member of the American Economic Association, the Population Association of America, and the Gerontological Society of America. She has a B.A. in economics from the University of Wisconsin and an honorary Sc.D. from the College of Medicine and Dentistry of New Jersey. Her major interests include health statistics, the impact of an aging population, cost of illness studies, and the economics of medical care.

CAROLYN C. ROGERS, who served as research associate during the first year of the study, is currently a research associate with Child Trends, Inc., in Washington, D.C. At the time of the study, she was on leave to the panel from the Bureau of the Census. Her major research interests include fertility, delayed childbearing, and child care arrangements; she has published numerous articles and reports on fertility-related issues, many based upon analyses of the Census Bureau's Current Population Survey. She is a member of the Population Association of America. She received an M.A. degree in sociology/demography from Brown University.

JOHN W. ROWE, a geriatrician, is director of the Division on Aging at Harvard Medical School, chief of gerontology at Beth Israel and Brigham and Women's Hospitals, and director of the Veterans Administration's Boston-area Geriatric Research Education Clinical Center. A recipient of a B.S. degree from Canisius College and an M.D. from the University of Rochester, he was trained in internal medicine at Beth Israel and Massachusetts General Hospitals and in gerontology at the National Institute on Aging. His research focuses on the physiological changes accompanying normal aging and their clinical impact. His past service on national committees includes chairmanship of the National Institutes of Health study section on aging. He is currently chairman of the Institute of Medicine's project on Leadership for Geriatric Medicine and the MacArthur Foundation Research Program on Successful Aging.

ETHEL SHANAS is professor emerita of sociology and professor emerita of health care services at the University of Illinois at Chicago. She received B.A., M.A., and Ph.D. degrees in sociology from the University of Chicago. In 1985 she received an honorary degree of doctor of humane letters from Hunter College, City University of New York. She is a past president of the Gerontological Society of America and of the Midwest Sociological Society and the 1986 chair of the section on aging of the American Sociological Association. As a member of the National Committee on Vital and Health Statistics, she served as chair of the consultant panel that developed the Long-Term Health Care Minimum Data Set. She is a senior member of the Institute of Medicine.

JAMES H. WARE is professor of biostatistics at the Harvard School of Public Health. He received a B.A. in mathematics from Yale University and a Ph.D. in statistics from Stanford University. He spent eight years at the National Heart, Lung, and Blood Institute before joining the Harvard faculty in 1979. His research interests include statistical methods for longitudinal studies, epidemiologic methods, and statistical aspects of environmental research.